Brief Con

Preface   xi

CHAPTER 1 **Practices of Intravenous Therapy   1**

CHAPTER 2 **Safety and Infection Control   21**

CHAPTER 3 **Intravenous Therapy Supplies and Equipment   39**

CHAPTER 4 **Intravenous Fluids, Components, and Compatibility   69**

CHAPTER 5 **Preparation and Patient Communication   99**

CHAPTER 6 **Monitoring and Maintaining Intravenous Therapy   130**

CHAPTER 7 **Documenting and Discontinuation   152**

CHAPTER 8 **Intravenous Therapy Calculations   172**

APPENDIX A **Intravenous Fluid Abbreviations and Concentrations   201**

APPENDIX B **Incompatible Intravenous Medications and Solutions   203**

APPENDIX C **Common Intravenous Medications   204**

APPENDIX D **Conversions, Abbreviations, and Formulas for Intravenous Calculations   206**

APPENDIX E **Answer Key   208**

APPENDIX F **Competency Checklists   219**

Glossary   228

Credits   233

Index   235

Contents

Preface   xi

CHAPTER 1   **Practices of Intravenous Therapy   1**

   I. Introduction   2
   II. IV Therapy Practice and Regulation   3
   III. Roles and Responsibilities   5
      a. Allied Health Personnel   6
      b. Medical Assistants   6
   IV. Reasons for IV Therapy   7
      a. Maintaining Fluid and Electrolyte Balance   7
         i. Electrolytes   8
         ii. Fluid Movement   9
         iii. Other Fluid Regulation Processes   9
      b. Administering Medications   10
      c. Administering Blood and Blood Products   10
      d. Delivering Nutrients and Nutritional Supplements   12
   V. Types of IV Therapy   13
      e. Peripheral IV Therapy   13
      f. Central IV Therapy   14
         i. Peripherally Inserted Central Catheter (PICC)   15
         ii. Central Venous Lines   16
         iii. Implantable Ports   16

CHAPTER 2   **Safety and Infection Control   21**

   I. Introduction   22
   II. Standards for Safe-Needle and Needleless Devices   22
   III. Safe-Needle Devices   24
   IV. Needleless Systems   26
         i. Blunt Cannula and Resealable Ports   26
         ii. Luer-Activated Devices (LADs)   27
         iii. Pressure-Activated Safety Valve Devices   27
   V. Infection Control   28
      a. The Chain of Infection   29
         i. Links in the Chain of Infection   29
         ii. Modes of Transmission   30
      b. Preventing Infections   30
   VI. Hand Hygiene   32
         i. Personal Protective Equipment (PPE)   33

INTRAVENOUS THERAPY

FOR HEALTH CARE PERSONNEL

Kathryn A. Booth, RN-BSN, MS, RMA

Total Care Programming

 Higher Education

Boston   Burr Ridge, IL   Dubuque, IA   New York   San Francisco   St. Louis
Bangkok   Bogotá   Caracas   Kuala Lumpur   Lisbon   London   Madrid   Mexico City
Milan   Montreal   New Delhi   Santiago   Seoul   Singapore   Sydney   Taipei   Toronto

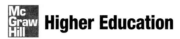

Higher Education

INTRAVENOUS THERAPY FOR HEALTH CARE PERSONNEL

Published by McGraw-Hill, a business unit of The McGraw-Hill Companies, Inc., 1221 Avenue of the Americas, New York, NY 10020. Copyright © 2008 by The McGraw-Hill Companies, Inc. All rights reserved. No part of this publication may be reproduced or distributed in any form or by any means, or stored in a database or retrieval system, without the prior written consent of The McGraw-Hill Companies, Inc., including, but not limited to, in any network or other electronic storage or transmission, or broadcast for distance learning.

Some ancillaries, including electronic and print components, may not be available to customers outside the United States.

♻ This book is printed on recycled, acid-free paper containing 10% postconsumer waste.

2 3 4 5 6 7 8 9 0 QPD/QPD 0 9 8

ISBN 978–0–07–340193–5
MHID 0–07–340193–5

Publisher: *Michelle Watnick/David Culverwell*
Senior Sponsoring Editor: *Roxan Kinsey*
Developmental Editor: *Connie Kuhl*
Senior Marketing Manager: *Nancy Bradshaw*
Senior Project Manager: *Sheila M. Frank*
Senior Production Supervisor: *Sherry L. Kane*
Lead Media Project Manager: *Audrey A. Reiter*
Interior Design: *Laurie B. Janssen*
Cover Design: *Studio Montage*
 (USE) Cover Image: *©Gettyimages/Medicine Today V59*
Senior Photo Research Coordinator: *Lori Hancock*
Photo Research: *LouAnn K. Wilson*
Compositor: *Precision Graphics*
Typeface: *10.5/13 Melior*
Printer: *Quebecor World Dubuque, IA*

The credits section for this book begins on page 233 and is considered an extension of the copyright page.

Library of Congress Cataloging-in-Publication Data

Booth, Kathryn A., 1957—
    Intravenous therapy for health care personnel / Kathryn A. Booth. — 1st ed.
        p. cm
    Includes index.
        ISBN 978–0–07–340193–5 — ISBN 0–07–340193–5 (alk. paper)
        1. Intravenous therapy. I. Title.

RM170
615'.6—dc22

2006052748

Dedication

To the individuals who are learning intravenous therapy and who are meeting the needs of the health care workforce. May your careers be rewarding and satisfying as you provide this technical care to patients in need.

This book is, as always, also dedicated to my best friend, husband, and partner, Jim, who has made my life dreams a reality.

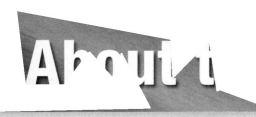

Kathryn A. Booth, RN-BSN, MS, RMA, is a full-time author, educator, and consultant for Total Care Programming, a multimedia software development company. Her background includes a bachelor's degree in nursing and a master's degree in education. Her 27 years of teaching, nursing, and health care work experience spans four states. She has authored and developed multimedia software and health care textbooks and educational materials for McGraw Hill Higher Education; Total Care Programming; Glencoe/McGraw-Hill; Mosby Lifeline; and Lippincott, Williams, and Wilkins. Kathy has presented at numerous state, corporate, and national conventions since 1994. Her current focus is to develop up-to-date, dynamic health care education materials to assist educators and promote the health care profession. To remain current, Kathy has most recently worked as a part-time LPN instructor and a practicing medical assistant, and she has just completed her RMA certification.

CHAPTER 3 **Intravenous Therapy Supplies and Equipment 39**

    I. Introduction 40
   II. Catheters and Access Devices 40
      a. Peripheral Access Devices 41
         i. Needle and Syringe 41
        ii. Over-the-Needle Catheter 42
       iii. Steel Needle 43
      d. Needleless Systems 44
         i. Midline Peripheral Catheters and Peripherally Inserted Central Catheters 44
        ii. Central Venous Catheters 46
       iii. Centrally Placed External Catheters 46
       iv. Centrally Placed Internal Ports 48
  III. Venous Access Device Selection 49
      a. Factors to Consider 50
      b. Catheter Sizes 50
  IV. Administration Equipment 51
      a. Primary Administration Sets 52
      b. Secondary Administration Sets 54
      c. Accessory Devices for IV Administration 55
   V. Fluids 57
  VI. IV Regulators 59
      a. Manual Monitoring 59
      b. Infusion Pumps 60
      c. Rate Controllers 61
      d. Syringe Pumps 61
      e. Patient-Controlled Analgesia Pumps 61
      f. Volume-Control Sets 62

CHAPTER 4 **Intravenous Fluids, Components, and Compatibility 69**

    I. Introduction 70
   II. Types and Uses of IV Fluids 72
      a. Sodium Chloride Solutions 75
      b. Dextrose Solutions 75
      c. Solutions with a Combination of Sodium Chloride and Dextrose 75
      d. Multiple Electrolyte Solutions 76
      e. Plasma Expanders 76
      f. Blood and Blood Products 77
         i. ABO Blood Groups 77
        ii. Rh Factor 79
       iii. Blood Transfusions 80
  III. Additives 80
      a. Parenteral Nutrition 80
      b. Heparin 82
      c. Insulin 83
      d. Electrolytes and Vitamins 83
  IV. Compatibility 85

V. Common IV Medications 86
   a. Classification of Medications 87
      i. Anti-infectives 89
      ii. Cardiovascular Medications 90
      iii. Central Nervous System Medications 90
      iv. Gastrointestinal Medications 91
      v. Chemotherapeutic Agents 91
   b. Administration of IV Medications 92

CHAPTER **Preparation and Patient Communication 99**

I. Introduction 100
II. Preparation for the IV Infusion 101
   a. Physician's Orders 101
   b. Patient Preparation 102
      i. Psychological Preparation 103
      ii. Physical Preparation 103
III. Patient Identification and Screening 105
   a. Screening before an IV infusion 105
   b. Screening and Monitoring during IV Administration 106
IV. Site Selection for Peripheral IVs 107
   a. Site Selection 107
   b. Peripheral Veins 108
      i. Digital Dorsal Veins 110
      ii. Dorsal Metacarpal Veins 111
      iii. Cephalic Vein 111
      iv. Accessory Cephalic Vein 111
      v. Basilic Vein 111
      vi. Median Cephalic and Median Basilic Veins 111
      vii. Median Antebrachial Vein 111
      viii. Other Sites 111
V. Preparation of Supplies and Equipment 112
VI. Initiation of Peripheral IV Therapy 116
VII. Special Populations 122
   a. Geriatric Patients 122
   b. Obese Patients 123
   c. Pediatric Patients 123
      i. Immobilization 123
      ii. Venipuncture Sites 124

CHAPTER **Monitoring and Maintaining Intravenous Therapy 130**

I. Introduction 131
II. Labeling 131
   a. Site Label 131
   b. Rate Label 133
   c. Pharmacy Label 134

   III. Site Dressings and Changes 136
      a. Caring for the IV Site 136
      b. Changing the Dressing 137
   IV. Complications and Risks 138
      a. Infiltration 139
      b. Extravasation 140
      c. Phlebitis 141
      d. Other Complications 143
   V. Common Problems and Solutions 145
      a. IV Access 145
      b. Flow Rates 145
      c. IV Removal Problems 147

CHAPTER 7 **Documenting and Discontinuation 152**

   I. Introduction 153
   II. Documenting IV Therapy 153
      a. Documentation after IV Initiation 153
      b. Documentation during IV Therapy 154
      c. Documentation after IV Discontinuation 154
      d. Abbreviations in Documentation 155
   III. Monitoring IV Therapy 158
   IV. Documenting Fluid Balance 161
      a. Intake and Output 161
      b. Documenting Fluids 162
   V. Discontinuing an IV 165

CHAPTER 8 **Intravenous Therapy Calculations 172**

   I. Introduction 173
   II. Calculating Flow Rates 173
      a. Calculating Flow Rates in Milliliters per Hour (mL/h) 174
        i. Using the Formula Method 174
        ii. Using Dimensional Analysis 175
      b. Calculating Flow Rates in Drops per Minute (gtt/min) 176
        i. Using the Formula Method 177
        ii. Using Dimensional Analysis 178
   III. Adjusting Flow Rates 181
   IV. Calculating Infusion Time and Volume 184
      a. Calculating Infusion Time 184
        i. Using the Formula Method 184
        ii. Using Dimensional Analysis 185
      b. Calculating Infusion Volume 188
        i. Using the Formula Method 188
        ii. Using Dimensional Analysis 189

V. Calculating Intermittent Infusions   191
   a. Secondary Lines (Piggyback)   191
   b. Intermittent Peripheral Infusion Devices   191
   c. Preparing and Calculating Intermittent Infusions   192

Appendix A   Intravenous Fluid Abbreviations and Concentrations   201
Appendix B   Incompatible Intravenous Medications and Solutions   203
Appendix C   Common Intravenous Medications   204
Appendix D   Conversions, Abbreviations, and Formulas for Intravenous Calculations   206
Appendix E   Answer Key   208
Appendix F   Competency Checklists   219
Glossary   228
Credits   233
Index   235

Preface

The health care field today is in critical need of skilled professionals to care for patients who require intravenous (IV) therapy for diagnostic and therapeutic purposes. *Intravenous Therapy for Health Care Personnel* is your one-of-a-kind, just-in-time resource for the theory and basics of IV therapy, including entry-level skills such as IV preparation, monitoring, and maintenance and IV initiation and discontinuation. Whatever nursing or allied health profession you are interested in, you will find that this easy-to-use text/workbook/CD has the content to meet your professional needs. This resource accommodates self-paced study, traditional classroom use, or distance learning and is presented in multiple learning styles to ensure that your journey through *Intravenous Therapy for Health Care Personnel* will be a perfect fit.

The text/workbook/CD is divided into eight chapters.

- Chapter 1, Practices of Intravenous Therapy, introduces you to the field of IV therapy and discusses roles, responsibilities, organizations, and laws related to IV therapy. You also learn the reasons for and types of IV therapy.

- Chapter 2, Safety and Infection Control, addresses the standards that are set for IV therapy, including safe-needle and needleless devices. In addition, this chapter describes the necessary practices to prevent infection.

- In Chapter 3, Intravenous Therapy Supplies and Equipment, you learn about the various supplies and equipment needed for IV therapy, including catheters and access devices, administration equipment, and IV regulators.

- Chapter 4, Intravenous Fluids, Components, and Compatibility, introduces you to the types of fluids and additives that are part of IV therapy, including IV medications. Compatibility of these fluids and additives is another essential topic of this chapter.

- Chapter 5, Preparation and Patient Communication, helps you develop the knowledge and skills necessary for preparing the patient, the supplies, and the equipment for IV therapy. Also addressed are site selection, patient identification, considerations for special populations, and the theory and procedure for initiating an IV.

- Chapter 6, Monitoring and Maintaining Intravenous Therapy, explains the labeling process and the procedure for site dressing changes. You also learn about the complications and risks of IV therapy as well as common problems and solutions.

- The essential skills of documenting IV therapy is covered in detail in Chapter 7, Documenting and Discontinuation, including documentation after IV initiation, during IV therapy, and after discontinuation. Monitoring IV therapy, maintaining fluid balance, and discontinuing an IV are other topics presented in this chapter.
- The final chapter, Intravenous Therapy Calculations, presents the knowledge you need for calculating and adjusting flow rates and for understanding infusion time and volume as well as intermittent infusions and medications.

Features of the Text/Workbook/CD

- **Key Terms, Glossary, and Audio Glossary:** Key terms are identified at the beginning of each chapter. These terms are in **bold** type within the chapter and are defined both in the chapter and in the glossary at the end of the book. Open the student CD to hear the pronunciation of each key term, and practice learning the term with the Key Term Concentration game.
- **Checkpoint Questions:** At the end of each main heading in the chapter are short-answer Checkpoint Questions. Answer these questions to make sure you have learned the basic concepts presented.
- **CD Activities:** After you have finished the Checkpoint Questions, you are sent to the interactive student CD activity to further your review and practice of the concepts presented in each section. Be sure to complete the activities on the CD before you continue to the next section.
- **Troubleshooting:** The troubleshooting feature identifies problems and situations that may arise when you are caring for patients or performing a procedure. At the end of this feature, you are asked a question to answer in your own words.
- **Safety and Infection Control:** You are responsible for providing safe care and preventing the spread of infection. This feature presents tips and techniques to help you practice these important skills relative to IV therapy.
- **Patient Education and Communication:** Patient interaction and education and intrateam communication are integral parts of health care. As part of your daily duties, you must communicate effectively both orally and in writing and must provide patient education. Use this feature to learn ways to perform these tasks.
- **HIPAA, Law, and Ethics:** When working in health care, you must be conscious of the regulations of HIPAA (Health Insurance Portability and Accountability Act) and understand your legal responsibilities and the implications of your actions. You must perform duties within established ethical practices. This feature helps you gain insight into how HIPAA, law, and ethics relate to the performance of your duties.
- **Chapter Summary and Review:** Once you have completed each chapter, take time to read the summary and complete the chapter review questions, which are presented in a variety of formats. These questions help you understand the content presented in each chapter.

- **Get Connected and the Online Learning Center:** The Get Connected activity directs you to the Online Learning Center (OLC) that accompanies the text/workbook. The OLC provides links for you to complete research and activities relative to the information presented in the chapter. You will also find other review activities and materials on the OLC to assist you in learning IV therapy.
- **Chapter Test:** Open the student CD to take a final test of your knowledge relative to each chapter. Review the material again with the Spin the Wheel game and then take the chapter test. You can print or e-mail your score to your instructor.

Instructor's Manual and Instructor CD

Look to the Instructor's Manual and the Instructor CD for multiple resources to use while teaching *Intravenous Therapy for Health Care Personnel*. PowerPoint presentations for each chapter have Apply Your Knowledge questions at the end of each section and can be used for classroom presentation and discussion. An *EasyTest* test bank that contains a variety of questions with graphics allows you to simply and easily create your own final or chapter exam. Also available are suggested classroom activities that will increase the interest level and comprehension of the text/workbook/CD material. Anticipatory set activities for each chapter help stimulate and enhance student learning as you begin each new topic. Curriculum suggestions provide information on how to use the materials based on your course length and depth. All media on the student CD are conveniently provided on the instructor CD for classroom presentations.

Guided Tour

Chapter Outlines, Learning Outcomes, Key Terms, and an Introduction begin each chapter to introduce you to the chapter and help prepare you for the information that will be presented.

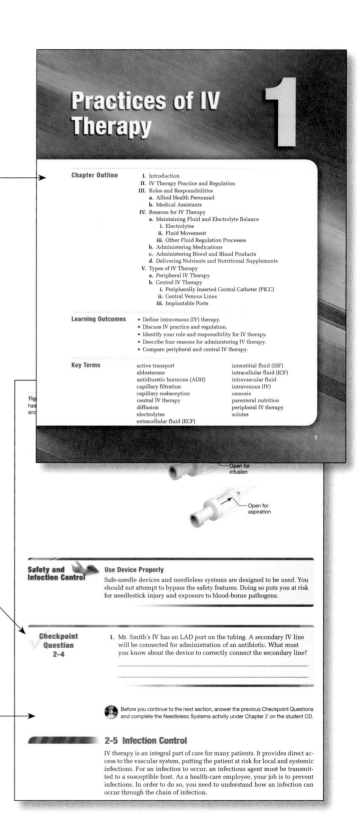

Practices of IV Therapy — 1

Chapter Outline
I. Introduction
II. IV Therapy Practice and Regulation
III. Roles and Responsibilities
  a. Allied Health Personnel
  b. Medical Assistants
IV. Reasons for IV Therapy
  a. Maintaining Fluid and Electrolyte Balance
    i. Electrolytes
    ii. Fluid Movement
    iii. Other Fluid Regulation Processes
  b. Administering Medications
  c. Administering Blood and Blood Products
  d. Delivering Nutrients and Nutritional Supplements
V. Types of IV Therapy
  a. Peripheral IV Therapy
  b. Central IV Therapy
    i. Peripherally Inserted Central Catheter (PICC)
    ii. Central Venous Lines
    iii. Implantable Ports

Learning Outcomes
• Define intravenous (IV) therapy.
• Discuss IV practice and regulation.
• Identify your role and responsibility for IV therapy.
• Describe four reasons for administering IV therapy.
• Compare peripheral and central IV therapy.

Key Terms
active transport
aldosterone
antidiuretic hormone (ADH)
capillary filtration
capillary reabsorption
central IV therapy
diffusion
electrolytes
extracellular fluid (ECF)
interstitial fluid (ISF)
intracellular fluid (ICF)
intravascular fluid
intravenous (IV)
osmosis
parenteral nutrition
peripheral IV therapy
solutes

Open for infusion

Open for aspiration

Safety and Infection Control   **Use Device Properly**
Safe-needle devices and needleless systems are designed to be *used*. You should not attempt to bypass the safety features. Doing so puts you at risk for needlestick injury and exposure to blood-borne pathogens.

Checkpoint questions are provided at the end of each section in the chapter to help you understand the information you just read.

Checkpoint Question 2-4
1. Mr. Smith's IV has an LAD port on the tubing. A secondary IV line will be connected for administration of an antibiotic. What must you know about the device to correctly connect the secondary line?

Before you continue to the next section, answer the previous Checkpoint Questions and complete the Needleless Systems activity under Chapter 2 on the student CD.

CD-ROM references direct you to the interactive CD activity to further your review and practice the concepts presented in each section.

2-5 Infection Control

IV therapy is an integral part of care for many patients. It provides direct access to the vascular system, putting the patient at risk for local and systemic infections. For an infection to occur, an infectious agent must be transmitted to a susceptible host. As a health-care employee, your job is to prevent infections. In order to do so, you need to understand how an infection can occur through the chain of infection.

Troubleshooting exercises identify problems and situations that may arise on the job. You may be asked to answer a question about the situation.

Patient Education and Communication boxes give you helpful information communicating effectively—both orally and written—with patients.

"I felt the chapters were well organized and very comprehensive and I actually learned some factual information myself from reviewing the contents."—Gerry Brasin, CMA, AS, CPC—Premier Education Group

pointed up. Use at least one towel to remove the majority of moisture and discard. Obtain another paper towel to ensure the hands are throughly dry. Use a dry paper towel to turn off the faucet if necessary. For routine hand washing, you can use a nonantimicrobial soap. Use an antimicrobial soap during a specific outbreak of infection. When using an alcohol-based hand rub, make sure you have no visible dirt or contamination on your hands. Apply a small amount (3 to 5 mL or ½ to 1 tsp) of the cleanser onto one hand, and rub your hands together vigorously until dry. Make sure all surfaces of your hands and fingers are covered. Alcohol-based hand rubs decontaminate the hands faster than washing, are better at killing bacteria, and are not as drying as soaps. Many health-care facilities have hand cleansers mounted outside each patient or exam room to facilitate hand hygiene.

Troubleshooting   **Using Proper Hand Hygiene**

You are changing a very soiled dressing on a patient's IV access site. Just as you finish, the patient's lunch tray arrives and you must clean your hands prior to assisting him with his meal.

Both soap and water and an alcohol-based hand rub are available. How do you decide which to use?

_____
_____
_____

Patient Education & Communication   **Help Patients Understand Infection Control Measures**

Some patients may feel as though you think they are "dirty" when they see you engaging in proper infection control procedures such as hand hygiene and gloving. Explain to patients the principles of infection control. Your explanation will make them aware of the reasons for hand hygiene and the use of gloves and will help them prevent infections at home and in the health-care environment.

Personal Protective Equipment (PPE)

In addition to hand washing, **personal protective equipment** such as gloves, gowns, masks, and eye protection can help prevent the spread of infection. Gloves provide a protective barrier, prevent contamination of the hands, reduce the risk of exposure to blood-borne pathogens, and prevent the spread of pathogens to and from patients and other health-care workers (Figure 2-7).
CDC recommendations for the use of gloves include

- Removing gloves and washing hands after any activity that contaminates the gloves/hands
- Changing gloves between patients
- Changing gloves during the care of a single patient when moving from one procedure to another, such as bathing the patient and then performing IV site care
- Using disposable gloves only once

An IV pole is another accessory device for IV infusion. These poles are used alone or with an electronic infusion pump. IV poles are typically on wheels for easy movement. Some IV poles are attached directly to the bed or stretcher.

Safety and Infection Control   **Maintain a Closed IV System**

An IV that is attached to a patient and in progress is called a closed system. When an IV line is breeched (opened)—to add accessory devices, for example—it creates an entry port for infection. Ideally, you should add accessory devices such as filters, stopcocks, connectors, and adaptors to the IV system before you connect the IV to the patient. If you must add accessory devices after the infusion has begun, use strict aseptic technique to prevent contamination of the system.

Safety and Infection Control boxes present tips and techniques for you to apply on the job.

Checkpoint Questions 3-4

1. What are the differences between a macrodrip administration set and a microdrip one?

_____
_____

2. When should a secondary administration set be used?

_____
_____
_____

Before you continue to the next section, answer the previous Checkpoint Questions and complete the Administration Equipment activity under Chapter 3 on the student CD.

3-5 Fluids

Most IV fluids come in soft, flexible plastic containers, although glass containers may be used for certain medications (Figures 3-21 and 3-22). IV fluid bags can hold solution amounts that range from 50 mL to 2000 mL, but they most often contain 500 or 1000 mL of solution. Smaller bags of fluid (50 to 250 mL) are usually used for IV medications (Figure 3-23). All IV bags are labeled with their contents by the manufacturer. Some IV bags include an injection port so that additional medication can be added to the solution. The amount of fluid that a patient receives is considered part of that patient's intake and must be recorded. When you are infusing IV fluid into a patient, you will follow specific guidelines for monitoring and recording this information at regular intervals. See Chapters 6 and 7 for more information about monitoring and documenting IV fluid intake.

Plastic IV fluid bags are sometimes covered with a transparent plastic wrap that must be removed before administration. If the pharmacist has added medication to the solution, the plastic wrap may already be removed. In either case, check the IV fluid bag for leaks or punctures. Also, check the

HIPAA, Law & Ethics

Follow HIPAA Guidelines

Always chart all information in the appropriate places on the patient's written or electronic medical record, and remember to sign and/or record your documentation. Do not leave completed charts or monitors in sight of patients or visitors. Doing so is a violation of patient confidentiality and HIPAA regulations.

Patient Education & Communication

Ensuring Accurate Intake and Output

When intake and output recording is required during IV therapy, all measurements must be accurate. Stress to the patient as well as to the patient's family and visitors the importance of measuring the patient's intake and output. Provide education to family members who may feel that they are helping when they empty a urinal or bedpan. Instruct the patient to call you after using the bedpan or urinal so that you can measure the output amount. If the patient is ambulatory and able to use the toilet, instruct the patient to place the urine collection container under the toilet seat to collect the urine to be measured (Figure 7-4). Remind the patient and visitors that no one but the patient should drink from the water pitcher or consume fluids from the meal tray, that doing so could lead to erroneous information about the patient's fluid balance.

HIPAA, Law, and Ethics boxes help you gain insight into necessary information related to the performance of your duties.

Chapter Summary

- The flow rate for an electronic infusion device is calculated in milliliters per hour. For a manually controlled IV or when an electronic device needs to be checked, the flow rate is calculated in drops per minute.
- If the IV flow rate is too fast or too slow, it should be adjusted. The new flow rate is calculated from the amount of solution left in the bag and the time remaining for the infusion. The percentage or amount of adjustment is regulated by the facility; typically, the adjustment does not exceed 25 percent of the original flow rate.
- Sometimes the physician's order gives only the infusion rate and the volume of fluid to infuse. The duration, or amount of time the IV will take to infuse, must be calculated in order that the IV can be properly monitored.
- In some situations, the physician's order for an IV gives only the duration and the flow rate. For proper administration, the volume of fluid to be infused must be calculated.
- The three steps for administering intermittent medications are (1) reconstitute the medication, (2) calculate the amount to administer, and (3) calculate the flow rate.

Key points in the Chapter Summaries help you review what was just learned.

Chapter Review

Chapter Reviews consist of various methods of quizzing you. True/False, Multiple Choice, Matching, and Critical Thinking questions appeal to all types of learners.

At the end of each chapter, you will be directed to visit the Internet and the student CD to experience more interactive activities about the information you just learned.

"This is a great introductory text for our Medical Assisting program. It covers all the aspects of IV therapy at a level that our students could comprehend."—David Rice, AA, BA—Career College of Northern Nevada

Matching

_____ 1. pathogen
_____ 2. virulence
_____ 3. Standard Precautions
_____ 4. susceptible host
_____ 5. personal protective equipment
_____ 6. nosocomial infection
_____ 7. chain of infection
_____ 8. reservoir
_____ 9. mode of transmission
_____ 10. isolation precautions

a. person at risk for infection
b. source of a pathogen
c. group of six steps that lead to infection
d. how a pathogen is spread
e. ability of a pathogen to cause disease
f. precautions taken with all patients to prevent the spread of infection
g. infectious agent
h. steps taken to prevent the spread of specific infections
i. equipment designed to protect the user
j. an infection acquired in the hospital

True/False

T F **11.** Needlestick injuries expose health-care workers to blood-borne pathogens such as HIV and hepatitis B and C viruses.
T F **12.** Health-care workers have no personal responsibility to prevent needlestick injuries.
T F **13.** Failure to activate safe-needle features puts the user at risk for needlestick injury.
T F **14.** Standard Precautions are used only with patients who have specific infections.
T F **15.** Washing your hands or using an alcohol-based hand rub is the best way to prevent the spread of infection.

Multiple Choice

16. How can needlestick injuries be prevented?
a. proper education and training
b. safer equipment
c. eliminating needles when possible
d. all of the above

Acknowledgm

Many thanks to the consultants Susan, Roberta, and Patti and reviewers who helped make this project complete. Their time, efforts, and expertise are greatly appreciated. A special thanks to Connie Kuhl, for the hard work and positive attitude. She is truly the nucleus of this project and a pleasure to work with as always. To Lori Hancock for dealing with the figure changes and Sheila Frank who kept the project going even with our delivery issues.

Consultants

Susan Hurley Findley, RN, MSN
Houston, TX

Roberta Pavy Ramont Ed.D, R.N
Seal Beach, CA

Patricia Dei Tos, RN, MSN, WPD
Fairfax, VA

Reviewers

Jason Amich, MSc, Medical
    Program
*Indiana Business College,
    Fort Wayne, IN*

Gerry Brasin, CMA, AS, CPC
*Premier Education Group,
    Springfield, MA*

Karen Brown, RN, EdD, Associate
    Dean of Instruction
*Kirtland Community College,
    Roscommon, MI*

Christina Rauberts Conklin, AA,
    RMA
*Florida Metropolitan University
    Tampa, FL*

Mary Dey, CMA-AC
*Kalamazoo Valley Community
    College, Kalamazoo, MI*

Carol Dravet
*Brown Mackie College,
    Merrillville, IN*

Melissa L. Dulaney
*MedVance Institute of Baton Rouge,
    Baton Rouge, LA*

Lynn M. Egler, RMA, AHI
*Virginia Career Institute,
    Virginia Beach, VA*

Tammy Gant, CMA, RHIT, CAHI
*Surry Community College,
    Dobson, NC*

Kathleen L. Garza, RN, MS, FNP
Hocking College, Nelsonville, OH

Cheri Goretti
*Quinebaug Valley Community
    College, Danielson, CT*

Jonathan Greenwald
*Arapahoe Community College,
    Littleton, CO*

Kris Hardy, CMA
*Brevard Community College,
    Cocoa, FL*

Chris Hollander, CMA, MA
*Westwood College-Denver North,
    Denver, CO*

Carol Lee Jarrell, MLT, AHI
*Brown Mackie College,
    Merrillville, IN*

Cathy Kelley-Arney, BSHS, CMA
*National College of Business and
    Technology, Bluefield, VA*

Robin Kerns, R.N., BSN, Medical
  Assisting Program Director
*Moultrie Technical College,
  Moultrie, GA*

Karmon L. Kingsley, CMA, CHI
*Cleveland State Community College,
  Cleveland, TN*

David O. Martinez
*Southwest Career Institute,
  El Paso, TX*

David Rice, AA, BA
*Career College of Northern Nevada,
  Reno, NV*

Sara Jones Wallace, C.RS
*Miller-Motte Technical College,
  Wilmington, NC*

Jay Wilborn
*National Park Community College,
  Hot Springs, AR*

Practices of IV Therapy

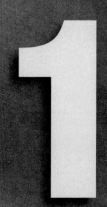

Chapter Outline

I. Introduction
II. IV Therapy Practice and Regulation
III. Roles and Responsibilities
    a. Allied Health Personnel
    b. Medical Assistants
IV. Reasons for IV Therapy
    a. Maintaining Fluid and Electrolyte Balance
       i. Electrolytes
       ii. Fluid Movement
       iii. Other Fluid Regulation Processes
    b. Administering Medications
    c. Administering Blood and Blood Products
    d. Delivering Nutrients and Nutritional Supplements
V. Types of IV Therapy
    a. Peripheral IV Therapy
    b. Central IV Therapy
       i. Peripherally Inserted Central Catheter (PICC)
       ii. Central Venous Lines
       iii. Implantable Ports

Learning Outcomes

- Define intravenous (IV) therapy.
- Discuss IV practice and regulation.
- Identify your role and responsibility for IV therapy.
- Describe four reasons for administering IV therapy.
- Compare peripheral and central IV therapy.

Key Terms

active transport
aldosterone
antidiuretic hormone (ADH)
capillary filtration
capillary reabsorption
central IV therapy
diffusion
electrolytes
extracellular fluid (ECF)

interstitial fluid (ISF)
intracellular fluid (ICF)
intravascular fluid
intravenous (IV)
osmosis
parenteral nutrition
peripheral IV therapy
solutes

1-1 Introduction

Intravenous (IV) simply means "within a vein." IV therapy is a treatment that infuses fluids, medications, blood, or blood products into a vein for treatment of a patient (Figure 1-1). It permits accurate dosing and a swift effect of the substance infused. IV therapy is used to administer fluids, drugs, and nutrients when a patient cannot take these items orally. The rapid effect of fluids delivered directly into the bloodstream is necessary during emergencies or other critical-care situations in which medications are needed. However, the results can be fatal if the wrong medication or dosage is given.

Current IV therapy is less than 100 years old. Yet, it was known as early as the 1600s that medications could be injected into a vein. Because of a lack of understanding about sterility, infection control, and other scientific methods, original attempts to deliver IV fluids and drugs met with little success. The greatest advance in drugs, equipment, and procedures has occurred in the past 25 years. The practice and regulation surrounding IV therapy continues to evolve.

Checkpoint Questions 1-1

1. Why would an IV be started?

_____

_____

2. When are patients most likely to have an IV?

_____

_____

Figure 1-1 Intravenous therapy is used to deliver fluids, drugs, or nutrients directly into a vein.

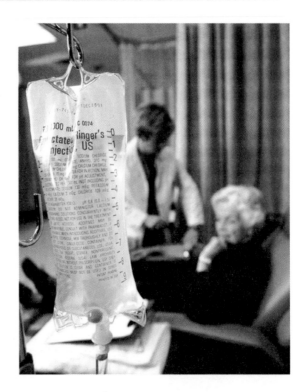

1-2 IV Therapy Practice and Regulation

The practice of IV therapy is closely controlled by laws and monitored by various organizations. Each institution or agency where you are employed will have specific policies guided by these laws and organizations. These organizations include the Joint Commission on Accreditation of Healthcare Organizations (JCAHO), Health Insurance Portability and Accountability Act (HIPAA), Centers for Disease Control and Prevention (CDC), National Institute of Occupational Safety and Health (NIOSH), and the Occupational Safety and Health Administration (OSHA).

JCAHO, the organization responsible for the accreditation of health care facilities, establishes the National Patient Safety Standards. These standards are updated yearly, and several of them apply to the practice of IV therapy. Table 1-1 identifies the selected goals that could apply to IV therapy.

HIPAA is a federal law passed in 2003 that protects the privacy and confidentiality of patient information. Among other provisions, HIPAA states that information about a patient must not be discussed with individuals other than the patient unless the patient has given written or verbal permission for you to do so. The following is a list of other guidelines from HIPAA that could apply to the care of patients with an IV infusion.

- Close patients' room doors when caring for them or discussing their health.
- Do not talk about patients in public places.
- Turn computer screens that contain patient information so passersby cannot see the information.
- Log off computers when you are done.
- Do not walk away from patient medical records; close them when leaving.

Look for more information and guidelines related to HIPAA in the feature boxes throughout this textbook.

CDC, an agency of the federal government, works to prevent and control infectious and chronic diseases, injuries, workplace hazards, disabilities, and environmental health threats. CDC collects information about infections that occur because of IV therapy. This information is used to track the source of infections and help prevent them.

NIOSH, a division of CDC, conducts research and makes recommendations for the prevention of work-related illnesses and injuries. Through their research into needlestick injuries, NIOSH has recommended that health care facilities use safer medical devices to protect workers from needlestick and other sharps injuries.

OSHA, as a division of the Department of Labor, has the responsibility of protecting the safety of employees in their place of employment. OSHA's mission is to ensure the safety and health of workers by setting and enforcing standards; providing training, outreach, and education; establishing partnerships; and encouraging continual improvement in workplace safety and health. OSHA has established universal and standard precautions along with the updated blood-borne pathogen standard, all of which prevent infection and injuries to health care workers.

Through the recommendation of NIOSH and the efforts of OSHA, the Needlestick Safety and Prevention Act was passed into law in 2001. The intent of the new law and the implementation regulation is to mandate the use

TABLE 1-1 National Patient Safety Standards (Selected Goals As They Pertain to IV Therapy)

Goal	Description	Comment
Goal 1. Improve the accuracy of patient identification.	1A. Use at least two patient identifiers (neither to be the patient's room number) whenever administering medications or blood products, taking blood samples and other specimens for clinical testing, or providing any other treatments or procedures.	*Before any IV therapy procedure is performed on a patient, the patient should be properly identified by at least two identifiers (neither of which should be the patient's room number).*
Goal 2. Improve the effectiveness of communication among caregivers.	2A. For verbal or telephone orders or for telephonic reporting of critical test results, verify the complete order or test result by having the person receiving the order or test result read back the complete order or test result.	*IV therapy orders or laboratory results should be read back to verify their accuracy.*
	2B. Standardize a list of abbreviations, acronyms, and symbols that are to be used throughout the organization.	*Use only abbreviations, acronyms, and symbols that are standardized by your health care facility.*
	2C. Measure, assess, and, if appropriate, take action to improve the timeliness of the reporting of critical test results and values and the timeliness of receipt of this information by the responsible licensed caregiver.	*Report test results regarding IV therapy to the licensed caregiver as soon as possible.*
Goal 3. Improve the safety of using medications.	3B. Standardize and limit the number of drug concentrations available in the organization.	*Check the concentrations of medications carefully to ensure that the proper medication is used.*
	3C. Identify and, at a minimum, annually review a list of look-alike/soundalike drugs used in the organization, and take action to prevent errors involving the interchange of these drugs.	*Check all medications at least three times to ensure that the correct medication is used.*
Goal 7. Reduce the risk of health care–associated infections.	7A. Comply with current Centers for Disease Control and Prevention (CDC) hand hygiene guidelines.	*Wash your hands before and after every procedure. Approved antiseptic hand rubs may be used if no visible soilage is on your hands.*
Goal 8. Accurately and completely reconcile medications across the continuum of care.	8A. Implement a process for obtaining and documenting a complete list of the patient's current medications upon the patient's admission to the organization and with the involvement of the patient. This process includes a comparison of the medications that the organization provides to those on the list.	*Ensure that all medications are recorded completely and accurately.*
	8B. A complete list of the patient's medications is communicated to the next provider of service when a patient is referred or transferred to another setting, service, practitioner, or level of care within or outside the organization.	*Ensure that a complete list of medications is provided for the patient when he or she receives service from another physician or health care facility.*

Source: Adapted from the Joint Commission on Accreditation of Healthcare Organizations, www.jcaho.org

of safety devices that reduce needlestick injuries in the clinical setting. OSHA can now impose monetary fines on any health care facility that is not using an appropriate safety IV catheter. These devices are discussed in Chapter 2, Safety and Infection Control. Additional information about safety and infection control related to IV therapy can be found in the features throughout this textbook.

Checkpoint Questions 1-2

1. What organizations and laws regulate the practice of IV therapy?

   _____

   _____

2. What is being done to reduce the incidence of needlestick injuries?

   _____

   _____

3. Which organization sets the standards of practice to prevent infection during IV therapy?

   _____

   _____

 Before you continue to the next section, answer the previous Checkpoint Questions and complete the IV Therapy Practice and Regulation activity under Chapter 1 on the student CD.

1-3 Roles and Responsibilities

An order for IV therapy is made by the physician. Various other health care employees are responsible for the procedures surrounding initiation, administration, and maintenance of the IV therapy that has been ordered. Each profession's role and responsibility are regulated by that profession's scope of practice, training, and state of practice and by the organization or facility of practice. By reading this textbook, you are preparing to learn the principles of IV therapy, which is one of the first requirements to practicing IV therapy. However, even after successfully completing this course, you will need to be aware of *your* scope of practice as well as your state regulations and the policies of the facility at which you are working.

Never perform any of the procedures in this textbook without first determining if the procedure is within your scope. It is your responsibility to know the laws that regulate your actions and also to consider your knowledge and experience when deciding whether you should perform the procedure. Keep in mind the difference between invasive and noninvasive procedures. Invasive procedures, such as starting or flushing an IV, carry with them additional dangers to the patient and typically require additional specialized training. Noninvasive procedures, such as setting up the IV equipment and monitoring or discontinuing an IV, carry less risk to the patient. Depending on your position and place of employment, both invasive and noninvasive procedures may be part of your scope and training.

Allied Health Personnel

Because of downsizing, restructuring, and nursing shortages in many areas of the country, various tasks of IV therapy may be performed by allied health personnel other than by registered nurses (RNs), such as licensed practical nurses (LPNs), licensed vocational nurses (LVNs), patient-care technicians (PCTs), and medical assistants (MAs). When performing IV therapy tasks, LPNs or LVNs must have the necessary preparation and experience. In addition, they must be authorized by their employer and by the state in which they work before they perform any procedures. LPNs and LVNs are governed by the Nurse Practice Act in their state and are accountable for any procedure they accept and perform. PCTs, depending on their training and place of employment, may be trained to set up the equipment to start an IV or to monitor the IV while it is in place.

Medical Assistants

Medical assistants mostly perform noninvasive procedures during IV therapy. Their tasks may include preparation, monitoring, maintenance, and documentation of IV therapy. In some circumstances, they may assist a physician or other licensed personnel during invasive procedures. In all cases the Medical Assistant practices under the direction and supervision of a licensed physician or other licensed health care practitioner. Because of this expanded role, the revised Commission on Accreditation of Allied Health Education Programs (CAAHEP) Standards and Guidelines for Medical Assisting Educational Programs indicates that accredited programs must include the principles of IV therapy. In some states, medical assistants are specifically forbidden from doing IV procedures. In other states, they are allowed if they meet certain requirements. In most states, the law is not clear as to whether a physician may delegate IV procedures to a medical assistant.

In order to prepare for the certified medical assistant (CMA) examination of the American Association of Medical Assistants (AAMA), you must know and understand the theory of IV therapy. More importantly, whether you are a registered medical assistant (RMA) or a CMA, you should be aware of the scope of practice within your state regarding IV therapy. Research the laws in your state to determine what procedures you may or may not perform. Many potential complications are associated with the use of IV therapy, and practicing outside your scope could result in injury to the patient and in possible malpractice lawsuits.

Troubleshooting **Determining Your Role**

You have moved into a new state and have begun work at a same-day surgery clinic. Because of the shortage of health care employees, you are placed with a postoperative patient your first day. The patient is ready to leave, and the physician asks you to remove the patient's IV before he leaves. You have had training and have removed several IVs at your previous place of employment.

How would you determine what to do?

_____

_____

1. If you are asked to perform a particular procedure that you have not been trained to do, what should you do?

_____

_____

2. What procedure relative to IV therapy is considered invasive?

_____

_____

3. What noninvasive IV therapy procedures are more commonly performed by entry-level allied health personnel?

_____

_____

Before you continue to the next section, answer the previous Checkpoint Questions and complete the Roles and Responsibilities activity under Chapter 1 on the student CD.

1-4 Reasons for IV Therapy

The most common reasons that a physician may order IV therapy for a patient include:

- To replace and maintain fluid and electrolyte balance
- To administer medications, including chemotherapeutic agents, intravenous anesthetics, and diagnostic reagents
- To transfuse blood and blood products
- To deliver nutrients and nutritional supplements

Maintaining Fluid and Electrolyte Balance

In an adult weighing 155 lb (70 kg), about 60 percent of the total body weight is fluid. In an infant, fluids account for about 80 percent of the total body weight. Body fluids are composed of water and **solutes,** which are dissolved

Figure 1-2 Body fluids are located in various compartments separated by cell membranes.

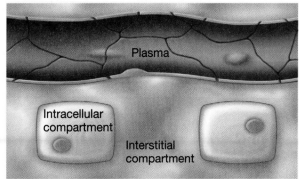

substances. Solutes include electrolytes, such as potassium, and nonelectrolytes, such as proteins. Body fluids have the following purposes:

- Help regulate body temperature
- Transport nutrients around the body
- Transport wastes to excretion sites
- Preserve cell shape

Body fluids are located in compartments. These compartments are separated from each other by cell membranes. The intracellular compartment holds the **intracellular fluid (ICF)**, or fluid inside the cell. Intracellular fluid comprises about 55 percent of total body fluid. **Extracellular fluid (ECF)**, or the fluid outside the cells, is found in the interstitial compartment (between and around cells) and the intravascular compartment (inside the blood vessels). **Interstitial fluid (ISF)**, which is the fluid that surrounds the cells, is in the interstitial compartment. **Intravascular fluid**, or blood plasma, the liquid component of the blood, is found in the intravascular compartment. ECF makes up about 45 percent of the total body fluid, and about 5 percent of ECF is intravascular fluid (Figure 1-2).

The body's fluid balance is regulated by hormones and is affected by fluid volume, distribution of fluids in the body, and concentration of solutes in the fluid itself. Each day the body gains fluids by oral intake through liquids and water in foods. It loses fluids through respiration, perspiration, urine, and feces. Gains must equal losses to maintain the body's fluid balance. A patient who is ill may have fluid volume depletion due to the inability to eat or drink or due to vomiting, diarrhea, and/or diaphoresis (sweating). This patient may require IV therapy.

Electrolytes

Electrolytes are chemicals that separate into electrically charged particles (ions) that conduct electricity necessary for normal cell function. Electrolytes are either positively charged ions, called cations, or negatively charged ions, called anions. Ions are not distributed evenly throughout the intracellular and extracellular fluids because of the cell membranes that separate the ICF and ECF. The cell membranes are selectively permeable and allow only certain ions to cross into or out of the cell. Although the ICF and ECF contain different solutes, the amount of these solutes is about equal when balance is maintained.

The six major electrolytes in body fluids are

1. Sodium
2. Potassium
3. Calcium
4. Chloride
5. Phosphate
6. Magnesium

Of these, potassium and phosphorus are the major intracellular electrolytes, and sodium and chloride are the major extracellular electrolytes. Potassium and sodium are cations, and phosphorous and chloride are anions. The ECF components—interstitial fluid and intravascular fluid—have the same electrolyte compositions; therefore, electrolytes can move freely between the two, keeping an equal distribution in both compartments.

Fluid Movement

Fluid and electrolyte balance is also regulated by fluid movement. Body fluids continually move among the major fluid compartments. In addition to regulating fluid and electrolyte balance, this constant movement permits nutrients, waste products, and other substances to move into and out of cells. Fluid movement is affected by cell membrane permeability and by concentrations of solutes in the fluid. When solutes and fluids are equal on both sides of the membrane, balance is maintained. Normally, the body can restore an imbalance by moving solutes and fluids across the cell membranes as necessary by one of several methods: diffusion, active transport, osmosis, capillary filtration, and reabsorption.

Solutes move across cell membranes by either diffusion or active transport. **Diffusion,** a passive process that requires no energy, is the most frequent process for movement of solutes. Diffusion moves solutes from an area of higher concentration across a membrane to an area of lower concentration and results in equal distribution of solutes between compartments. **Active transport** requires energy to move solutes from an area of lower concentration across a membrane to an area of higher concentration.

Osmosis, capillary filtration, and reabsorption are the methods that move fluids across membranes. **Osmosis** is a passive process in which water or other fluid simply moves from an area of higher concentration across a membrane to an area of lower concentration. Osmosis is dependent on the concentration of solutes in the fluid compartments and stops when concentrations on both sides of the membrane are equal. **Capillary filtration** forces fluid and solutes through the capillary wall pores from the intravascular fluid into the interstitial fluid. **Capillary reabsorption** keeps capillary filtration from removing an excess of intravascular fluid.

Other Fluid Regulation Processes

In addition to the fluid and electrolyte movements within the cells, the body maintains internal balance through the renal, cardiovascular, respiratory, and endocrine systems. The kidneys (renal system) control fluid and electrolyte balance by retaining or excreting urine as well as excreting metabolic wastes and toxic substances. The heart and blood vessels circulate blood through the kidneys, making urine output possible, and assist in fluid regulation by way of fluid volume and pressure sensors. Lungs remove water from the body during exhalation. The endocrine system produces hormones that regulate fluid volume and concentration. **Antidiuretic hormone (ADH)** from the pituitary gland regulates water retention. The hormone **aldosterone** from the adrenal glands causes the retention of sodium when the circulating fluid volume is low, when the sodium level is low, or the potassium level is high.

Thirst also regulates water volume and participates in maintaining fluid balance. A person becomes thirsty when water loss equals 2 percent of the body weight or when solute concentration increases. The drinking of water or other liquids reestablishes plasma volume and dilutes solute concentration. When a patient cannot replace lost fluids orally, IV solutions become necessary to help the patient maintain fluid and electrolyte balance.

Monitoring IV Therapy

Children (pediatric patients) have a larger percentage of fluid in their bodies than do adults. Mature adults (geriatric patients) may have conditions that compromise their fluid and electrolyte balance. For these reasons, it is more difficult to maintain the fluid and electrolyte balance in pediatric and geriatric patients. Both these types of patients will require very careful monitoring during IV therapy.

Administering Medications

Approximately 40 percent of the medications administered in the inpatient setting are given intravenously. Medications introduced directly into the bloodstream produce the rapid results that are often necessary during emergencies, because the therapeutic levels of the medication are quickly reached. IV medications are typically added to solutions. Dosages are easily adjusted by changing the concentration of the medication in the solution or by changing the administration rate. If an adverse reaction occurs, administration can be stopped immediately, limiting the amount of medication absorbed. This rapid resolution is not possible with other routes of administration. The IV administration of medication is generally less painful for the patient than are subcutaneous (sub-Q) or intramuscular (IM) administrations because the IV route does not require frequent injections (Figure 1-3).

Figure 1-3 Intravenous medications are frequently administered from a second smaller container into the main intravenous infusion.

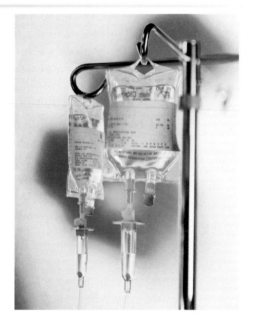

Administering Blood and Blood Products

Blood is the body's main transport system for oxygen, nutrients, hormones, and other important substances. Any decrease in the circulating volume disrupts the body's fluid and electrolyte balance. A patient who experiences a decrease in circulating blood volume may require replacement of blood or blood-based products (Figure 1-4).

Figure 1-4 When blood or blood products are administered, two health-care workers must check to be sure the correct match is made.

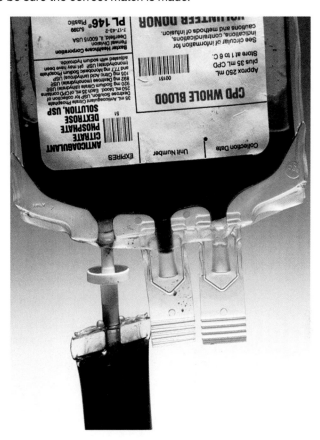

The process of blood transfusion takes blood or blood products from one individual and infuses the donated blood or blood products into the circulatory system of another individual. Blood transfusions are used to treat medical conditions such as blood loss due to trauma, surgery, shock, or failure of the mechanism that produces red blood cells (or some other normal and essential component). The infusion of blood or blood products restores circulating volume, improves the ability of the blood to carry oxygen, and replaces blood components that the body is deficient in, including factors that enable blood to clot.

Blood is made up of red blood cells, white blood cells, and platelets carried in plasma. To make the most use of donated blood, it is usually separated into components, and recipients may receive only parts of the blood. Blood transfusions typically consist of packed red blood cells rather than whole blood. White blood cell transfusions are less common. Plasma or platelets are given to patients with liver disease, cancer, severe burns, hemophilia, or leukemia because these components provide clotting factors.

When a patient is receiving blood or blood components, two health care workers must check the transfusion to be sure the correct match is made. Once the infusion is started, the patient's vital signs must be taken frequently in case of any reaction. Monitoring the vitals frequently and reporting any changes or abnormalities of the patient is mandatory. Most transfusions are performed without any problems. Mild side effects may include symptoms of an allergic reaction such as headache, fever, itching, increased breathing effort, or rash. Serious reactions are rare. The most common serious side effect is serum hepatitis, an infection of the liver. Transfusion with blood of the wrong type can be fatal, which is why many precautions are implemented throughout blood donation and during the transfusion of blood.

Delivering Nutrients and Nutritional Supplements

IV therapy can deliver some or all of the nutritional requirements for patients unable to obtain adequate amounts by oral or enteral (directly into the gastrointestinal tract) routes. **Parenteral nutrition** is the IV infusion of nutrients, including amino acids, dextrose, fat, electrolytes, vitamins, and trace elements (Figure 1-5). Parenteral nutrition solutions may be administered peripherally or through a central vein. Peripherally administered solutions are less concentrated and provide only partial nutritional requirements. Infusions through central veins can be more highly concentrated and, therefore, can provide the patient's total nutritional requirements.

Patient Education & Communication

Consent for IV Therapy

Before an IV is inserted into a patient, he or she must be educated about the procedure, including the reason and risks, and must agree either verbally or in writing.

Figure 1-5 Parenteral nutrition is the intravenous infusion of nutrients for patients who are unable to take adequate amounts by mouth or otherwise.

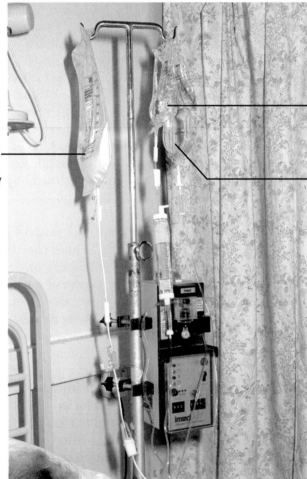

Fluids for parenteral nutrition are usually opaque.

This secondary IV may contain an antibiotic or other medication or additive.

Additional IV fluids are frequently administered with parenteral nutrition.

1. What are four reasons for IV therapy?

   _____

   _____

2. How does fluid movement occur in the cells?

   _____

   _____

3. What other processes regulate the fluid level in the body?

   _____

   _____

 Before you continue to the next section, answer the previous Checkpoint Questions and complete the Reasons for IV Therapy activity under Chapter 1 on the student CD.

1-5 Types of IV Therapy

IV therapy may be achieved by direct access of the vein with a syringe and needle, by a peripherally inserted catheter, or by a central IV catheter. All three are invasive procedures that require needle placement and administering the infusion or medication through an IV line or site.

Direct access of the vein is the simplest form of intravenous access. A syringe with an attached hollow needle is inserted through the skin into a vein, and the contents of the syringe are injected through the needle into the bloodstream. This method is most easily done with an arm vein, usually the antecubital vein at the crease of the elbow. The intravenous administration of medications provides no margin for errors; medications are often injected within one minute or less, so they reach the bloodstream immediately. Direct injection carries a higher risk for side effects and adverse reactions. Although it is a simple procedure, direct injection is rarely used because it allows delivery of only a single dose of medication.

Peripheral IV Therapy

Peripheral IV therapy is the preferred method for short-term IV therapy. It is the most common intravenous access method in hospitals, surgery centers, and paramedic services. A peripheral IV line consists of a short catheter (a few centimeters long) inserted through the skin into a peripheral vein. A peripheral vein is any vein that is not in the chest or abdomen. Arm and hand veins are typically used. Peripheral IV access is used for emergency care, for administration of medications and replacement fluids, and for blood or blood product infusions. Peripherally inserted catheters are easy to monitor and offer easy access to veins. However, peripheral veins frequently become inflamed from medications, or the IV infiltrates (that is, the IV solution infuses into surrounding tissue); both these problems necessitate removal and replacement at another site. (Infiltration of an IV is discussed in more

Figure 1-6   The back of the hand is commonly used for a peripheral IV site.

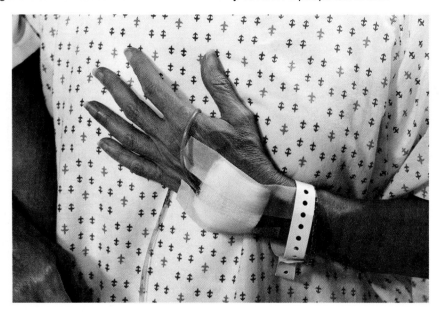

detail in chapter 6. Even if infiltration or inflammation does not occur, the peripheral catheter must be removed and a new catheter inserted at a different site every 72 hours. This necessary procedure will cause additional discomfort for the patient (Figure 1-6).

Central IV Therapy

Central IV therapy permits infusion of fluids or medications directly into a larger vein, usually the superior vena cava or within the right atrium of the heart. This method can be used in emergencies and permits venous access when a peripheral IV cannot be started. Central lines are used when a patient needs large volumes of fluids, long-term therapy, or multiple infusions. The advantages of central IV therapy are

- The ability to deliver fluids and medications that would be overly irritating to peripheral veins because of their concentration or chemical composition, such as some chemotherapy drugs and total parenteral nutrition
- Rapid onset of action because medications reach the heart immediately and are quickly distributed to the rest of the body
- Access to multiple parallel compartments (lumens) within the catheter, so that multiple medications can be delivered at the same time, even if they are chemically incompatible
- The ability to measure central venous pressure and other physiological variables

Because the IV is situated in a large central vein, it may also be used to obtain blood samples, and unless it becomes infected, it may remain in place for the duration of therapy, which decreases the number of venipunctures a patient must endure. Central IV lines carry higher risks of bleeding, bacteremia, and air embolism. These catheters require greater skill and time to insert and are more costly to maintain than are peripheral IV catheters.

Figure 1-7 Central IV therapy delivers fluids or medication directly into a larger vein for long-term, large-volume, or multiple infusions.

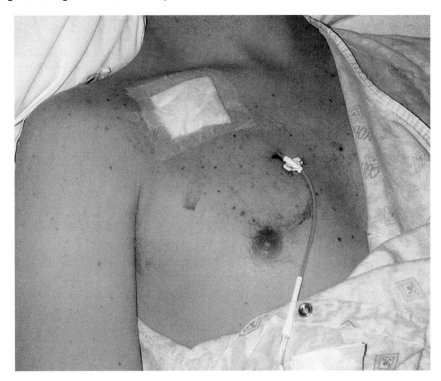

There are various types of central IV lines, but all must be inserted by a specially trained and licensed employee, usually the physician. It may be your responsibility to check these IV sites or monitor the infusion. Some central IV catheters are left in patients over long periods of time and are monitored in outpatient facilities (Figure 1-7).

Peripherally Inserted Central Catheter (PICC)

A peripherally inserted central catheter, or PICC, is inserted into a peripheral vein, usually in the arm, and then is carefully advanced upward until the catheter reaches the patient's superior vena cava or right atrium. Placement of the PICC is usually done by feel and estimation. An x-ray is then taken to verify that the tip is in the right place.

A PICC may have two parallel compartments, each with its own external connector (double lumen), or have a single tube and connector (single lumen). From the outside, a single-lumen PICC resembles a peripheral IV except that the tubing is slightly wider.

Because of the higher risk of infection, the PICC insertion site must be covered by a larger sterile dressing than would be required for a peripheral IV. However, a PICC poses less of a systemic infection risk than do other central IVs, because bacteria would have to travel up the entire length of the narrow catheter before spreading through the bloodstream.

The chief advantage of a PICC over other types of central lines is that it is easy to insert, poses a relatively low risk of bleeding, is externally unobtrusive, and can be left in place for months to years for patients who require extended treatment. The chief disadvantage is that it must travel through a relatively small peripheral vein, which means that the line is limited in diameter and is also somewhat vulnerable to occlusion or damage from movement or squeezing of the arm.

Central Venous Lines

Several types of catheters take a more direct route into central veins. These catheters are collectively called central venous lines. Physicians or other specially trained personnel usually insert central venous lines.

In the simplest type of central venous access, a catheter is inserted into a subclavian vein, an internal jugular vein, or (less commonly) a femoral vein and is advanced toward the heart until it reaches the superior vena cava or right atrium. In newborn infants, a central line can be inserted into the umbilical vein or artery. Because all these veins are larger than peripheral veins, central lines can deliver a higher volume of fluid and can have multiple lumens.

Another type of central line, called a Hickman or Broviac catheter, is inserted into the target vein and then "tunneled" under the skin to emerge a short distance away. This method reduces the risk of infection, because bacteria from the skin surface are not able to travel directly into the vein; also, these catheters are made of materials that resist infection and clotting.

Implantable Ports

A port (often referred to by brand names such as Port-A-Cath or MediPort) is a central venous line that does not have an external connector. Instead, it has a small reservoir implanted under the skin. Medication is administered intermittently by placing a small needle through the skin into the reservoir. Ports cause less inconvenience and have a lower risk of infection than do PICCs, and are therefore commonly used for patients on long-term intermittent treatment, such as chemotherapy.

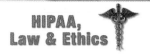
HIPAA, Law & Ethics

Patient Privacy

HIPAA, the Health Insurance Portability and Accountability Act, mandates that you protect the privacy of your patients' health information. HIPAA establishes punishments for anyone violating patient privacy. All information about any of your patients who require IV therapy must be kept private and confidential.

Checkpoint Questions 1-5

1. What are the two types of IV therapy?

   _____

   _____

2. Which type of central IV therapy would most likely be used for long-term IV chemotherapy on an outpatient basis?

   _____

   _____

Before you continue to the chapter summary, answer the previous Checkpoint Questions and complete the Types of IV Therapy activity under Chapter 1 on the student CD.

Chapter Summary

- IV therapy is a treatment that infuses fluids, medications, blood, or blood products into a vein for treatment of a patient. It involves both invasive and noninvasive procedures.
- Safety and the legal aspects of IV therapy are closely regulated by agencies and laws such as JCAHO, OSHA, CDC, NIOSH, and HIPAA.
- Your role and responsibility related to IV therapy is regulated by your training, the scope of practice of your profession, your state, your place of employment and the licensed physician or other licensed health care practitioner. Always know what you can and cannot do.
- The four most common reasons for IV therapy are to maintain fluid and electrolyte balance, to administer medications, to transfuse blood and blood products, and to deliver nutrients and nutritional supplements.
- Peripherally inserted catheters are used for short-term therapy; they provide easy access and are easy to monitor. Centrally inserted catheters are used for patients who need large volumes of fluids, long-term therapy, or multiple infusions.

Matching

_____ 1. interstitialfluid (ISF)

_____ 2. antidiuretic hormone (ADH)

_____ 3. parenteral nutrition

_____ 4. electrolytes

_____ 5. central IV therapy

_____ 6. aldosterone

_____ 7. intracellular fluid (ICF)

_____ 8. intravenous

_____ 9. extracellular fluid (ECF)

_____ 10. peripheral IV therapy

a. secreted from the adrenal glands and affects fluid balance

b. secreted from the pituitary gland and regulates the retention of water

c. infusion of fluids or medications directly into a large vein such as the superior vena cava

d. sodium, potassium, calcium, chloride, phosphorus, and magnesium

e. fluid outside the cells

f. fluid that surrounds the cells

g. fluid inside the cells

h. into a vein

i. infusion of nutrients including amino acids, dextrose, fat, electrolytes, vitamins, and trace elements

j. introduction of fluids through a catheter for short-term therapy

True/False

T   F   **11.** A patient may be put on IV therapy to replace fluid losses, receive medications, or receive transfused blood.

T   F   **12.** To discuss private information about a patient when the patient's door is open is a violation of HIPAA.

T   F   **13.** A peripheral IV access is preferred for long-term IV therapy.

T   F   **14.** Central IV lines deliver solutions and medications into large central veins, ensuring rapid onset of actions and rapid distribution to the rest of the body.

T   F   **15.** The medical assistant may perform preparation, monitoring, and maintenance of IVs in all states.

Multiple Choice

16. A patient has been vomiting for several days. Which of the following would the patient most likely be receiving?
    a. blood transfusion
    b. parenteral nutrition
    c. catheter
    d. an enema

17. The patient has cancer and will be receiving chemotherapy. Which of the following types of therapy would most likely be used?
    a. peripheral IV therapy
    b. direct injection
    c. central IV therapy
    d. physical therapy

18. Which of the following sets yearly standards for patient safety?
    a. HIPAA
    b. OSHA
    c. JCAHO
    d. CDC

19. Several patients at your facility who are receiving IV therapy develop a similar infection at the IV site. Which organization would track the cases of infection and help research the cause?
    a. OSHA
    b. JCAHO
    c. HIPAA
    d. CDC

20. Which of the following would be *unacceptable* if you are abiding by the guidelines set forth in HIPAA?
    a. signing out of the computer when leaving it
    b. talking to your supervisor about a patient in an occupied elevator
    c. turning the computer screen so people passing by cannot see it
    d. closing the room door when you speak with a patient

21. Which of the following is an invasive procedure related to IV therapy?
    a. starting an IV
    b. setting up the equipment for an IV
    c. discontinuing an IV
    d. monitoring an IV

22. Which of the following is the fluid that is found surrounding the cells?
    a. intercellular fluid
    b. extracellular fluid
    c. electrolytes
    d. interstitial fluid

23. Which of the following helps maintain fluid and electrolyte balance by regulating water retention?
    a. aldosterone
    b. active transport
    c. antidiuretic hormone (ADH)
    d. osmosis

24. Which of the following is considered an advantage of IV medication administration?
    a. It is more painful but also more effective.
    b. It can be stopped quickly when an adverse reaction occurs.
    c. It is given directly into a muscle during emergencies.
    d. It is given when the patient cannot take nutrition by mouth.

25. Which of the following is an advantage of peripheral IV therapy?
   a. Fluids and medication reach the heart immediately.
   b. The catheter may be used to administer chemotherapy.
   c. Multiple medications can be delivered at the same time.
   d. It is easy to monitor and access.

What Should You Do? (Critical Thinking/Application Questions)

1. When you take the equipment into a patient's room for an IV to be started, the patient asks, "What's that? What are you going to do?" What should you do?

_____

_____

_____

2. You receive a call about your patient named Carrie. The caller asks, "When did they put that IV in Carrie's arm? I just do not get it. I thought she was getting better. What happened? Why did the doctor order this IV?" What should you do?

_____

_____

_____

Get Connected

Visit the McGraw-Hill Higher Education website for *Intravenous Therapy for Health Care Personnel* at **www.mhhe.com/healthcareskills** to complete the following activities.

1. Use the Internet to research scope of practice in your state.
2. Visit the website of the Joint Commission on Accreditation of Healthcare Organizations (**www .jcaho.org**) and find the National Patient Safety Goals. Review the standards as they apply to the facility at which you will be employed. For example, if you work in ambulatory care, look for ambulatory-care standards.

Using the Student CD

Now that you have completed the material in Chapter 1, return to the student CD and complete any chapter activities you have not yet done. Practice your terminology with the Key Term Concentration game. Review the chapter material with the Spin the Wheel game. Take the final chapter test, complete the troubleshooting question, and e-mail or print your results to document your proficiency for this chapter.

Safety and Infection Control

2

Chapter Outline

    I. Introduction

    II. Standards for Safe-Needle and Needleless Devices

    III. Safe-Needle Devices

    IV. Needleless Systems

        i. Blunt Cannula and Resealable Ports

        ii. Luer-Activated Devices (LADs)

        iii. Pressure-Activated Safety Valve Devices

    V. Infection Control

      a. The Chain of Infection

        i. Links in the Chain of Infection

        ii. Modes of Transmission

      b. Preventing Infections

    VI. Hand Hygiene

        i. Personal Protective Equipment (PPE)

Learning Outcomes

- Compare and contrast needleless systems and safe-needle devices.
- Describe your responsibilities in the prevention of needlesticks.
- Discuss the purpose of hand hygiene.
- Relate CDC standards for hand hygiene to the practice of IV therapy.
- Perform hand hygiene before, during, and after IV therapy procedures.
- Identify when personal protective equipment is used during IV therapy.

Key Terms

airborne transmission	nosocomial infection
chain of infection	personal protective equipment
contact transmission	portal of entry
blood-borne pathogen	portal of exit
droplet transmission	reservoir
infectious agent	safe-needle devices
isolation precautions	Standard Precautions
mode of transmission	susceptible host
needleless systems	virulence
needlestick injuries	

2-1 Introduction

Safety and infection control are two very important elements for protecting both you and the patient when you are providing any aspect of IV therapy. The National Institute for Occupational Safety and Health (NIOSH) estimates that between 600,000 and 800,000 **needlestick injuries** occur annually, exposing health-care workers to **blood-borne pathogens** (microorganisms present in the blood that can cause disease) including human immunodeficiency virus (HIV), hepatitis C virus (HCV), and hepatitis B virus (HBV). A needlestick has both financial and emotional consequences. Follow-up for a high-risk exposure is approximately $500 to $1000 per needlestick even if no infection develops. However, the emotional impact and health consequences can be severe and can continue for a long time, especially if the exposure is to HIV. Needlestick injuries are preventable with proper education, safer equipment, and elimination of the need for needles whenever possible.

Another element of protection for health-care workers comes from infection control measures. Each year, approximately 1000 health-care workers contract serious infections from needlesticks and sharps exposure. Infection control measures also protect the patient from a hospital-acquired infection. The 2003 National Healthcare Quality Report found that approximately two infections per 1000 discharges occurred in the year 2003 because of intravenous lines or catheters. Although this seems like a small number, any hospital-acquired infection is unacceptable.

Checkpoint Question 2-1

1. What are the consequences of poor safety and infection control measures during IV therapy?

_____

_____

2-2 Standards for Safe-Needle and Needleless Devices

Safe-needle designs were first patented in the 1970s. More than 250 needle safety devices have now been approved for use. In 1992, the Food and Drug Administration recommended, but did not require, that health-care facilities use **needleless systems** for IV therapy. It was not until 2001, with passage of the Needlestick Safety and Prevention Act, that the use of **safe needle devices** was mandated and health-care facilities were required to use alternatives to needles whenever possible and to use devices with safety features when a needle was required. The introduction of needleless equipment and protected needles has significantly reduced the risk of needlestick injuries. All devices selected for IV therapy should be equipped with needlestick prevention features. Because of the Needlestick Safety and Prevention Act, health-care facilities are now required to

- Document the evaluation and implementation of safety-engineered sharp devices and needleless systems.
- Review and update exposure control plans at least annually to reflect changes in sharps safety technology.
- Maintain a sharps injury log.

- Include frontline health-care workers (actual users of the equipment) in the evaluation and selection process of safety-engineered sharp devices.
- Expand of the definition of *engineering controls* to include devices with engineered sharps injury protection. These controls (e.g., sharps disposal containers, self-sheathing needles, and needleless systems) should isolate or remove the blood-borne pathogens hazard from the workplace.

Even though your employer is obligated to provide the equipment and controls to reduce the possibility of needlestick injuries, you also have a responsibility to protect yourself and coworkers from needlestick injuries. You should

- Avoid the use of needles when possible
- Correctly use the safe alternatives provided
- Not recap needles
- Dispose of used needles promptly and in an appropriate sharps container
- Report hazards from needles that you observe in the workplace
- Report needlestick injuries promptly to ensure that you receive appropriate follow-up care
- Attend training and follow infection control policies and procedures

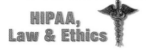

HIPAA, Law & Ethics

Reporting Needlestick Injuries

Whether you sustain a needlestick injury yourself or witness a coworker being stuck, you must report the injury to your supervisor. In addition, you are obligated to report hazards from needles that you observe in the workplace.

✓ Checkpoint Questions 2-2

1. What governmental act mandated that health-care facilities provide safer equipment to reduce the number of or prevent needlestick injuries?

   _____

   _____

2. What are your responsibilities in the prevention of needlestick injuries?

   _____

   _____

 Before you continue to the next section, answer the previous Checkpoint Questions and complete the Standards for Safe-Needle and Needleless Devices activity under Chapter 2 on the student CD.

2-3 Safe-Needle Devices

Most needlestick injuries occur during or after use and before disposal of the needle. These injuries are usually related to recapping needles and failing to dispose of used needles properly. Safe-needle devices are designed to decrease risks during all aspects of IV therapy. Many types of safe-needle devices are in use today. Ideally, such devices should

- Be needleless
- Have the needle built into the device
- Require no activation by the user (a passive device); if user activation is necessary, the safety feature should be activated without exposing the user to the sharp point and should easily enable the user to tell that it is activated
- Be easy to use and practical
- Be safe and effective for patient care

It is not always possible to use a completely needleless system. IV catheters and phlebotomy equipment require needles for ease of use. These catheters and needles have additional safety features to protect the health-care worker from accidental puncture with a contaminated needle. In most cases, the user is required to actively engage the safety feature. Table 2-1 provides examples of safe-needle devices.

When used correctly, safe-needle devices will reduce your risk of needlestick injury and exposure to blood-borne pathogens. *However, safety devices will only prevent injury when activated and when activated correctly.* Be sure to activate the safety feature as soon as the procedure is completed. Most devices are designed to be activated before the needle is removed from the patient or from the catheter. Failure to do so increases your risk. Keep your hands behind the exposed needle when activating the safety feature, and watch for the sign, such as an audible click or color change, that indicates the feature is engaged.

Checkpoint Questions 2-3

1. What is the purpose of safe-needle devices?

   _____

   _____

2. What precautions should you take when activating a safe-needle device?

   _____

   _____

 Before you continue to the next section, answer the previous Checkpoint Questions and complete the Safe-Needle Devices activity under Chapter 2 on the student CD.

TABLE 2-1 Safe-Needle Devices

Safety Feature	Example	Activation
Retractable needle		The needle is spring-loaded and retracts into the barrel. • Syringes with this feature are activated when the plunger is completely depressed following an injection. The needle may be fused to the syringe or be detachable. • IV catheters with this feature are activated by pushing a button (circled).
Protective sheath		The user slides a plastic cover over the needle and locks it in place. Both syringes and IV catheters can have this device.
Safety clip		The safety clip of a passive device is integrated into the catheter hub and is automatically engaged when the needle bevel exits the catheter hub.
Hinged-recap		A hinged protective cap flips down over the needle and locks into place. Needles with this feature may be fused to the syringe or be detachable.
Self-blunting needle		Needle is blunted after use. This device is generally used for blood collection. It requires the user to actively engage the feature by pushing the Vacutainer all the way into the holder or, in the case of a butterfly needle, flipping a wing to the side.

2-4 Needleless Systems

Needleless systems are the best systems to use because they eliminate the possibility of a needlestick injury (Figure 2-1). A needleless system generally includes the IV set and possibly an extension set. Secondary sets for infusing medications may also be a part of the system. (Specific IV therapy supplies and equipment are discussed in Chapter 3.) Some systems may require special cannulas for accessing ports. Needleless features are usually integrated into IV tubing, but add-on needleless ports are available to connect latex injection ports that are normally accessed with a needle. There are three types of needleless devices:

1. Blunt cannula and resealable ports
2. Luer-activated devices (LADs)
3. Pressure-activated safety valve devices

Blunt Cannula and Resealable Ports

The blunt cannula and resealable ports were components of the first needleless system introduced on the market. The blunt cannula attaches to a syringe or IV tubing (Figure 2-2). The device enables needleless IV access through a resealable port. The port is swabbed with an alcohol prep pad prior to insertion of the blunt cannula. It is important not to puncture this port with a needle because this compromises the integrity of the system. This

Figure 2-1 A needleless system like this one helps prevent needlestick injuries to health care workers and patients. A plunger and a special rubber stopper replace the needle.

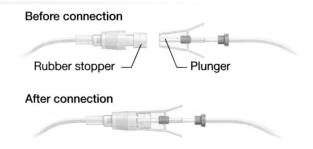

Before connection

Rubber stopper —   — Plunger

After connection

Figure 2-2 A blunt tip inserted into a resealable port is part of one type of needleless system.

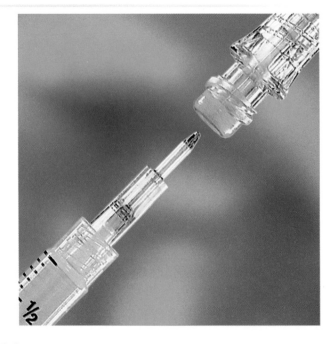

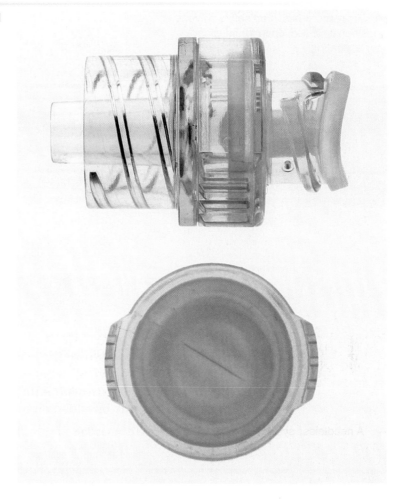

system is not as versatile as the Luer-activated device because of the need for a specialized tip on the syringe or tubing to access the port.

Luer-Activated Devices (LADs)

The two most common types of Luer-activated devices (LADs) are capped and capless (Figure 2-3). Both are antireflux valve ports and are activated when a standard syringe or IV set is connected to the port. They reseal when the syringe or tubing is removed. The capless port must be swabbed with an alcohol prep pad prior to use. The capped port is an older version of the LAD and requires capping with a sterile cap between uses to prevent contamination of the fluid pathway. LAD ports remain open until the syringe or tubing is removed. Because of this, blood can back up through these devices if the infusion runs dry or if it is used for intermittent IV access, such as a saline lock, and can result in catheter occlusion. The newest version of the LAD is the positive fluid displacement device, which is similar to the capless LAD for administration and flushing. This device expels a small amount of flush solution back into the catheter when disconnected, reducing the incidence of clotted catheters.

Pressure-Activated Safety Valve Devices

Pressure-activated safety valves have a slit silicone disk in the catheter hub. This device has three positions: closed, open forward for infusion, and open in the reverse direction for aspiration (Figure 2-4). The forward open position requires only a small amount of pressure for infusions. Because

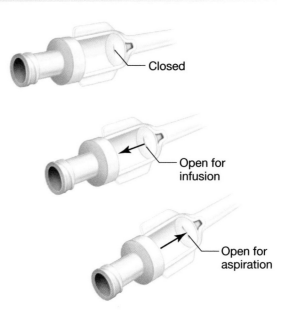

Figure 2-4 A pressure-activated safety valve has three positions: closed, open for infusion, and open for aspiration.

Closed

Open for infusion

Open for aspiration

the valve closes when pressure falls (such as when no solution is infusing), catheters cannot occlude when an unattended infusion runs dry. This device is most commonly used with central line catheters. It may be an integral part of the catheter, or it may be added on to the hub of any nonvalved catheter. The device can also be accessed by any standard syringe or IV tubing without special cannulas or other devices.

Safety and Infection Control

Use Device Properly

Safe-needle devices and needleless systems are designed to be *used*. You should not attempt to bypass the safety features. Doing so puts you at risk for needlestick injury and exposure to blood-borne pathogens.

Checkpoint Question 2-4

1. Mr. Smith's IV has an LAD port on the tubing. A secondary IV line will be connected for administration of an antibiotic. What must you know about the device to correctly connect the secondary line?

_____

_____

 Before you continue to the next section, answer the previous Checkpoint Questions and complete the Needleless Systems activity under Chapter 2 on the student CD.

2-5 Infection Control

IV therapy is an integral part of care for many patients. It provides direct access to the vascular system, putting the patient at risk for local and systemic infections. For an infection to occur, an infectious agent must be transmitted to a susceptible host. As a health-care employee, your job is to prevent infections. In order to do so, you need to understand how an infection can occur through the chain of infection.

The Chain of Infection

The **chain of infection** is six steps (links) that must take place for an infection to occur (Figure 2-5). The six links are the reservoir, infectious agent, portal of exit, mode of transmission, portal of entry, and susceptible host. Transmission of an infection can occur at any one of these six links in the chain of infection. Likewise, if the chain is broken at any of the links, an infection will not develop.

Links in the Chain of Infection

The first link of the chain of infection is the **infectious agent,** or pathogen itself. However, the presence of a pathogen does not always produce an infection. The body has many naturally occurring pathogens that under normal conditions do not cause infection. The ability of a pathogen to produce an infection depends on its **virulence** (ability to cause disease), the number of organisms or pathogens, the susceptibility of the host, and the presence of a portal of entry into the host.

The second link in the chain of infection is the **reservoir,** or source of the infectious agent. The reservoir is the site at which the organism grows and multiplies. It is most often a human or an animal. However, contaminated equipment may also be a reservoir for pathogens.

A **portal of exit** from the reservoir is the third link in the chain of infection. The pathogen must be able to move from the reservoir to the host. The major portals of exit from the human reservoir include the skin, respiratory tract, and gastrointestinal tract. Blood may also be a portal of exit and is a concern when you are performing IV therapy. If a patient's blood is infected, you are at risk of acquiring that infection.

Figure 2-5 If one of the links in the chain of infection is broken, infection can be prevented.

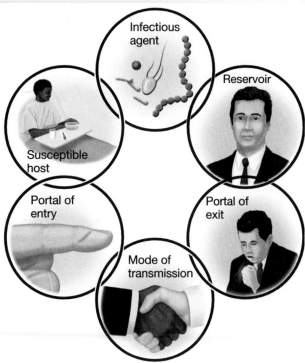

The fourth link in the chain of infection is the **mode of transmission**. The primary modes are contact, droplet, or airborne transmission. Transmission may also be *vehicle-borne*, from contaminated items such as equipment, food, or water, or *vector-borne*, from mosquitoes, rats, or fleas. The mode of transmission of an infectious agent determines the type of infection control protection you must use, which is discussed in the section titled Modes of Transmission.

The fifth link in the chain of infection is the **portal of entry**. An organism must be able to enter the body of a susceptible person to cause an infection. The skin is a good barrier against infection; however, any break in skin integrity, including an IV catheter, provides an entry point. The respiratory system is also a portal of entry. Most pathogens enter the host in the same way that they leave the source.

A **susceptible host** is the sixth link in the chain of infection. A person who is at risk to develop an infection when exposed to a pathogen is a susceptible host. A person becomes susceptible when natural defense mechanisms become impaired because of illness or age or even breaks in skin integrity, including IV catheters.

Modes of Transmission

Contact transmission is the most frequent source of **nosocomial infections** (infections acquired in a health-care facility) and can be by either direct or indirect contact. Direct contact requires a physical transfer of pathogens from reservoir to susceptible host (person to person) by something as simple as a touch. Indirect contact occurs when a contaminated item, such as a soiled dressing, is handled prior to contact with a susceptible host (person to contaminated item to person). Indirect contact most often occurs when healthcare workers fail to wash their hands and change gloves between patients. Methicillin-resistant *Staphylococcus aureus* (MRSA) and *Clostridium difficile* (C-diff) enteritis are examples of infections spread by contact transmission.

Droplet transmission is a form of contact transmission, but the method of transfer is much different. This form occurs when droplets from an infected person are propelled short distances to the susceptible host through the nasal mucosa, mouth, or conjunctiva. Examples of infections spread by droplet transmission are influenza, mumps, and rubella. Droplets are propelled by coughing, sneezing, breathing, or talking. The droplets are not suspended in the air, as they are with airborne transmission.

In **airborne transmission**, small particles carry the pathogens. These particles can be widely dispersed by air currents before being inhaled by a host. Legionnaires' disease, varicilla, and tuberculosis are examples of infections spread by airborne transmission.

Vehicle-borne transmission occurs when a host comes in contact with a contaminated item such as food, linen, or equipment. To prevent this mode of transmission, soiled linen and equipment must be cleaned or disposed of properly. Vector-borne transmission requires an animal or insect as an agent to spread disease, such as the mosquito that carries the West Nile virus.

Preventing Infections

Implementation of infection control measures can help prevent nosocomial infections in patients with impaired natural defenses and poor general health. Nosocomial infections occur while a patient is receiving care in a health-care facility; such infections are not present or incubating before the patient begins receiving the care. Nosocomial infections are caused directly by the health care that the patient receives.

To help prevent nosocomial infections, CDC in 1994 implemented two levels of precautions. The first level is **Standard Precautions.** These precautions combine hand hygiene and the wearing of gloves when health-care workers are exposed to blood and body fluids, nonintact skin, or mucous membranes. Standard Precautions include the major features of Universal Precautions, but they apply when workers are exposed to nonintact skin, mucous membranes, and blood and all body fluids, secretions, and excretions except sweat regardless of whether blood is visible. (Universal Precautions apply to blood and any other body fluids *only* if they contain visible blood.) The use of Standard Precautions reduces the risk of transmission of microorganisms from both recognized and unrecognized sources of infection. In addition, CDC advises that health-care workers should not wear artificial nails, because workers who wear artificial nails are more likely to harbor gram-negative pathogens on their fingertips than are workers with natural nails, both before and after hand washing. Natural nails should be no longer than one-fourth inch.

CDC's second level of precautions is **isolation precautions** that are based on how the infectious agent is transmitted. These isolation precautions are

- Airborne precautions that require special air handling, ventilation, and additional respiratory protection (HEPA or N95 respirators)
- Droplet precautions that require mucous membrane protection (goggles and masks)
- Contact precautions that require gloves and gowns during direct skin-to-skin contact or contact with contaminated linen, equipment, and so on

You should follow Standard Precautions with every patient when you are giving baths, changing dressings, emptying urinals or bedpans, and performing other routine care. Standard Precautions are essential during IV therapy procedures. Isolation precautions are used less often and only with patients who have specific infections. When isolation precautions are mandated for a patient receiving an IV, you will be required to follow the specific guidelines for the type of precautions implemented.

Checkpoint Questions 2-5

1. What is the chain of infection?

   _____

   _____

2. You are performing routine care for your assigned patient. What is the type of precautions that CDC recommends for care of an uninfected patient?

   _____

   _____

3. You must check the IV of a patient for whom airborne precautions have been implemented. What should you do?

   _____

   _____

Before you continue to the next section, answer the previous Checkpoint Questions and complete the Infection Control activity under Chapter 2 on the student CD.

2-6 Hand Hygiene

A health-care worker's hands carry many pathogens that are easily transferred to or from a patient or equipment and supplies during routine care. Hand hygiene is the simplest and most important way to prevent the spread of infection (Figure 2-6). CDC recommends that you wash your hands with soap and water whenever they are visibly contaminated with blood or other body fluids. If your hands are not visibly contaminated, they can be washed with soap and water or decontaminated with an alcohol-based hand rub. Wash your hands or use an alcohol-based hand rub in any of the following situations:

- Before and after direct contact with a patient and between patients
- Before putting on gloves (sterile or nonsterile) and after removing them
- After contact with body fluids or excretions, mucous membranes, non-intact skin, or wound dressings
- When moving from a contaminated body site to a clean body site during patient care
- After handling soiled linen, equipment, or supplies
- After sneezing or coughing
- Before and after eating
- After using the restroom

When washing your hands, keep your fingers pointed downward to prevent contamination of your arms; use soap from a dispenser; and do not touch any portion of the sink. Vigorously rub all surfaces for 10 to 15 seconds, starting at your fingers and moving toward your wrists. This motion produces friction that suspends the contaminants allowing them to be rinsed away. Dry your hands thoroughly with paper towels, keeping your fingers

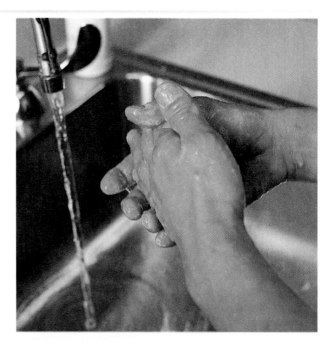

Figure 2-6 Hand washing is the single most important procedure to prevent the spread of infection.

pointed up. Use at least one towel to remove the majority of moisture and discard. Obtain another paper towel to ensure the hands are throughly dry. Use a dry paper towel to turn off the faucet if necessary. For routine hand washing, you can use a nonantimicrobial soap. Use an antimicrobial soap during a specific outbreak of infection. When using an alcohol-based hand rub, make sure you have no visible dirt or contamination on your hands. Apply a small amount (3 to 5 mL or ½ to 1 tsp) of the cleanser onto one hand, and rub your hands together vigorously until dry. Make sure all surfaces of your hands and fingers are covered. Alcohol-based hand rubs decontaminate the hands faster than washing, are better at killing bacteria, and are not as drying as soaps. Many health-care facilities have hand cleansers mounted outside each patient or exam room to facilitate hand hygiene.

Troubleshooting **Using Proper Hand Hygiene**

You are changing a very soiled dressing on a patient's IV access site. Just as you finish, the patient's lunch tray arrives and you must clean your hands prior to assisting him with his meal.

Both soap and water and an alcohol-based hand rub are available. How do you decide which to use?

_____

_____

Patient Education & Communication **Help Patients Understand Infection Control Measures**

Some patients may feel as though you think they are "dirty" when they see you engaging in proper infection control procedures such as hand hygiene and gloving. Explain to patients the principles of infection control. Your explanation will make them aware of the reasons for hand hygiene and the use of gloves and will help them prevent infections at home and in the health-care environment.

Personal Protective Equipment (PPE)

In addition to hand washing, **personal protective equipment** such as gloves, gowns, masks, and eye protection can help prevent the spread of infection. Gloves provide a protective barrier, prevent contamination of the hands, reduce the risk of exposure to blood-borne pathogens, and prevent the spread of pathogens to and from patients and other health-care workers (Figure 2-7).

CDC recommendations for the use of gloves include

- Removing gloves and washing hands after any activity that contaminates the gloves/hands
- Changing gloves between patients
- Changing gloves during the care of a single patient when moving from one procedure to another, such as bathing the patient and then performing IV site care
- Using disposable gloves only once

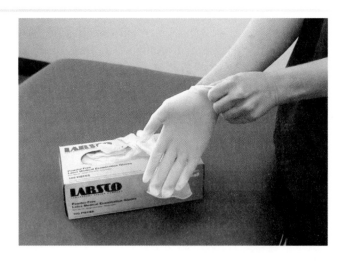

Figure 2-7 Gloves provide a protective barrier and are necessary during IV therapy, especially when the IV is started or discontinued.

Safety and Infection Control

Gloving Only is Not Enough

Wearing gloves does reduce the spread of infections; however, wearing gloves is not enough. Gloves are worn in addition to, not as a substitute for, hand washing.

Other types of personal protective equipment that may be part of Standard Precautions include gowns, masks, and eye protection. Nonsterile gowns protect skin and prevent contamination of clothing while you are providing patient care. To prevent the spread of infection, remove your gown immediately after you complete your task, and place it in an appropriate container.

To protect your eyes and mucous membranes from accidental exposure, wear a mask and eye protection such as goggles or a face shield when performing procedures that pose a risk of splashing blood and body fluids (Figure 2-8). Eyeglasses alone are not adequate protection because they do not fully cover the eyes; there are exposed spaces around the lenses. Goggles or face shields fully protect the eyes. If the patient has orders for either droplet or airborne isolation precautions, use a special mask such as the HEPA (high efficiency particulate air) filter or N95 mask.

Figure 2-8 A mask and eye protection should be worn when splashing or splattering of blood could occur.

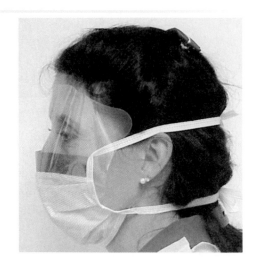

1. How does wearing gloves prevent the spread of infection?

_____

_____

2. You are assigned to check the IV of a patient who has tuberculosis. What type of personal protective equipment should you use?

_____

_____

 Before you continue to the chapter summary, answer the previous Checkpoint Questions and complete the Hand Hygiene activity under Chapter 2 on the student CD.

Chapter Summary

- Needlestick injuries expose health-care workers to blood-borne pathogens, including HIV, hepatitis C, and hepatitis B.
- Needleless and safe-needle devices decrease the risk for needlestick injuries.
- Health-care facilities are obligated to provide safer equipment, but health-care workers also have a responsibility to protect themselves and coworkers from needlestick injuries.
- The transmission of an infection agent can be prevented at any one of the six links in the chain of infection.
- Hand hygiene, including hand washing and the use of alcohol-based hand rubs, is the best way to prevent the spread of infection. Hand washing should be done when the hands are visibly soiled. Alcohol-based hand rubs can be used when no soil is visible.
- When using alcohol-based hand rubs or when washing your hands, vigorously rub your hands together, making sure to cover all surfaces.
- Personal protective equipment such as gloves, masks, or gowns help prevent the spread of infection by providing a protective barrier against contamination by blood and body fluids.

Matching

_____ **1.** pathogen

_____ **2.** virulence

_____ **3.** Standard Precautions

_____ **4.** susceptible host

_____ **5.** personal protective equipment

_____ **6.** nosocomial infection

_____ **7.** chain of infection

_____ **8.** reservoir

_____ **9.** mode of transmission

_____ **10.** isolation precautions

a. person at risk for infection

b. source of a pathogen

c. group of six steps that lead to infection

d. how a pathogen is spread

e. ability of a pathogen to cause disease

f. precautions taken with all patients to prevent the spread of infection

g. infectious agent

h. steps taken to prevent the spread of specific infections

i. equipment designed to protect the user

j. an infection acquired in the hospital

True/False

T   F   **11.** Needlestick injuries expose health-care workers to blood-borne pathogens such as HIV and hepatitis B and C viruses.

T   F   **12.** Health-care workers have no personal responsibility to prevent needlestick injuries.

T   F   **13.** Failure to activate safe-needle features puts the user at risk for needlestick injury.

T   F   **14.** Standard Precautions are used only with patients who have specific infections.

T   F   **15.** Washing your hands or using an alcohol-based hand rub is the best way to prevent the spread of infection.

Multiple Choice

16. How can needlestick injuries be prevented?
   a. proper education and training
   b. safer equipment
   c. eliminating needles when possible
   d. all of the above

17. Which of the following can you be exposed to as a result of a needlestick injury?
    a. HIV and hepatitis B and C
    b. tuberculosis
    c. measles, mumps, and rubella
    d. Legionnaires' disease and varicilla

18. Which of the following is *not* a link in the chain of infection?
    a. reservoir; mode of transmission
    b. isolation precautions
    c. portals of entry and exit
    d. susceptible host

19. How are pathogens transmitted?
    a. droplet, contact, or airborne transmission
    b. vector or vehicle transmission
    c. both a and b
    d. none of the above

20. How do you spread droplets that carry pathogens?
    a. changing a dressing without wearing gloves
    b. sneezing or coughing
    c. using contaminated equipment
    d. having contact with insects

21. A susceptible host is at risk for infection when which of the following is impaired?
    a. circulation of blood
    b. respiration
    c. mobility
    d. natural defense mechanisms

22. Which of these precautions should you take when performing routine patient care?
    a. Always wear a gown and mask during care.
    b. Wear gloves during care and wash hands after.
    c. Keep infected patients away from other patients.
    d. Only hand hygiene is necessary.

23. When should you wash your hands?
    a. before using the restroom
    b. following the use of an alcohol-based hand rub
    c. before and after direct contact with a patient
    d. only at the beginning of your shift

24. What governmental agency makes recommendations for hand hygiene?
    a. OSHA
    b. JCAHO
    c. HIPAA
    d. CDC

25. Why do you use personal protective equipment such as gowns and masks?
    a. to keep your uniform and your face clean
    b. to prevent the spread of infection to a patient
    c. to prevent the contamination of your clothes or mucous membranes during patient care
    d. to eliminate the need for hand hygiene

What Should You Do? (Critical Thinking/Application Questions)

1. You are assisting a coworker in changing the sheets and bathing a total-care patient who recently had an IV started. While removing the soiled linen, your coworker was stuck by an IV needle that had been left on the bed. She said that it was only a small stick and that she was not going to report it to her supervisor. What should you do?

   _____

   _____

   _____

2. You have just finished removing an IV from Mr. Gomez when his roommate, Mr. Johnson, tells you that he needs help off the bedpan "right now!" You still have on your gloves from removing the IV. What should you do?

   _____

   _____

   _____

Get Connected

Visit the McGraw-Hill Higher Education website for *Intravenous Therapy for Health Care Personnel* at **www.mhhe.com/healthcareskills** to complete the following activities.

1. You have been placed on a committee to help evaluate and recommend new safe-needle devices for your facility. First, determine the CDC-recommended guidelines for safe-needle devices by visiting their website (**www.cdc.gov**). Second, search the Internet for available devices. Write a brief summary of your findings.

2. Now that you have determined the requirements for safe-needle devices, the committee has asked you to research devices for IV therapy. Visit the website of the National Alliance for the Primary Prevention of Sharps Injuries (**www.nappsi.org**), review the available safe-needle devices for IV insertion, and select three devices to recommend to the committee. Write a brief summary describing the three devices you have selected.

Using the Student CD

Now that you have completed the material in Chapter 2, return to the student CD and complete any chapter activities you have not yet done. Practice your terminology with the Key Term Concentration game. Review the chapter material with the Spin the Wheel game. Take the final chapter test, complete the troubleshooting question, and e-mail or print your results to document your proficiency for this chapter.

Intravenous Therapy Supplies and Equipment

3

Chapter Outline

I. Introduction

II. Catheters and Access Devices
   a. Needle and Syringe
   b. Over-the-Needle Catheter
   c. Steel Needle
   d. Needleless Systems
   e. Other Intravenous Access Devices
      i. Midline Peripheral Catheters and Peripherally Inserted Central Catheters
      ii. Central Venous Catheters
      iii. Centrally Placed External Catheters
      iv. Centrally Placed Internal Ports

III. Venous Access Device Selection
   a. Factors to Consider
   b. Catheter Sizes

IV. Administration Equipment
   a. Primary Administration Sets
   b. Secondary Administration Sets
   c. Accessory Devices for IV Administration

V. Fluids

VI. IV Regulators
   a. Manual Monitoring
   b. Infusion Pumps
   c. Rate Controllers
   d. Syringe Pumps
   e. Patient-Controlled Analgesia Pumps
   f. Volume-Control Sets

Learning Outcomes

- Describe the various types of IV access devices.
- State the factors to be considered when selecting a venous access device.
- Identify common sizes of IV catheters and state their use.
- Discuss why the correct choice is always the shortest, smallest IV cannula that will accomplish the task.

- Compare primary and secondary administration sets.
- Explain the differences in drip rate between macrodrip and microdrip infusion sets.
- Summarize how IV therapy fluids are supplied.
- Differentiate among types of infusion rate control devices.

Key Terms

antecubital
cannula system
central venous line
electronic flow control device
extension tubing
heparin flush
infusion pump
injection cap
lumen
midline catheter
milliliter (mL)
patient-controlled analgesia (PCA)
   pump

peripheral vein
primary administration set
PRN adaptor
rate controller
saline flush
secondary administration set
stopcock
syringe pump
trocar
volume-control sets
Y set

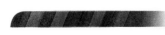

3-1 Introduction

In its early stages, IV therapy equipment comprised systems of glass bottles, hollow-bore metal needles, and manual control of gravity flow. Nowadays, the equipment has evolved to plastic fluid containers, electronic infusion pumps, and vein access devices that allow the needle to be removed, leaving only a polyethylene catheter in the vein. No matter what type of equipment is used or how basic or advanced the equipment is, the health care professional is still responsible for continuously monitoring the patient and the infusion to ensure that the physician's orders for the IV therapy are being carried out explicitly. This task requires knowledge of the supplies and equipment used for IV therapy.

Checkpoint Question 3-1

1. What is the health care professional's most important function when working with IV therapy?

_____

_____

3-2 Catheters and Access Devices

Catheters and access devices vary depending on the intended location and on the needs of the patient. Special devices are available for midline catheters, PICC lines, and central IV lines, but the most common devices are peripheral access devices (Figure 3-1).

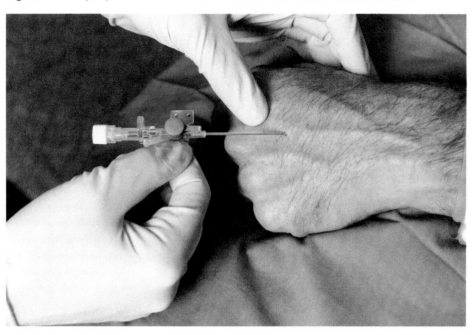

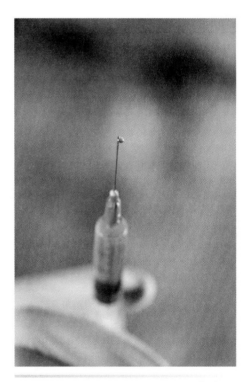

Figure 3-2   A syringe and needle device is used infrequently for IV access because only one dose of medication or fluid can be administered.

Peripheral Access Devices

Peripheral access devices are used to access the bloodstream through a **peripheral vein.** (A peripheral vein is any vein that is not in the chest or abdomen. Arm and hand veins are typically used.) Once a peripheral IV is established, a needleless system is used to infuse additional fluids or medications. The three main types of peripheral access devices are the needle and syringe, the over-the-needle catheter, and the steel needle.

Needle and Syringe

The simplest form of intravenous access is a syringe with an attached hollow needle (Figure 3-2). The needle is inserted through the skin into a vein, and the contents of the syringe are injected through the needle into the bloodstream. This procedure is most easily done with an arm vein, especially an **antecubital,** or vein on the inside of the elbow (e.g., the basilic or median cubical vein). It is necessary to use a tourniquet first, which makes the vein bulge and facilitates placement of the IV needle. Once the needle is in place, it is common to draw back slightly on the syringe until a blood return appears, thus verifying that the needle is really in a vein. The tourniquet is then removed prior to the injection. Although it is a simple procedure, direct injection is rarely used in a controlled health care setting because it only allows delivery of a single dose of medication.

Figure 3-3 An angiocath has a retraction button to prevent needlesticks when an IV is stated.

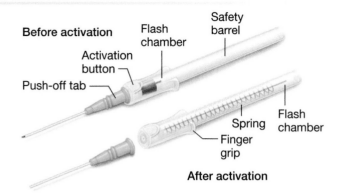

Before activation

Push-off tab

Activation button

Flash chamber

Safety barrel

Spring

Finger grip

Flash chamber

After activation

Over-the-Needle Catheter

An over-the-needle catheter has a needle inside a soft, flexible hollow tube (Figure 3-3). The needle pierces the skin, and then the soft catheter is held in place while the needle is removed. Part of the catheter remains outside the skin and has a hub that can be connected to a syringe or an IV infusion line or capped between treatments. One example of the over-the-needle catheter is the Angiocath system. The over-the-needle catheter is designed with a retraction button that, as soon as the catheter is advanced in the vein, can be pushed so that the needle is automatically shielded as it is removed; this design prevents needlesticks. Once the needle has been retracted, the introducer is removed and only the hollow plastic catheter remains in the vein. The administration set is attached to the hub, and the prescribed fluid is then infused. The over-the-needle catheter is the most common venous access device used in health care facilities because it meets the latest safety requirements and is more comfortable for the patient. The flexible cannula allows the patient more mobility.

A clear plastic dressing is normally placed over the catheter in order to keep it clean and dry at all times. Peripheral IV lines are designed to be used in settings in which they can be monitored and changed frequently; they are impractical for extended home use because of the potential for dislodging the small catheter from the vein. An active patient would have to be careful when moving about and performing daily activities. Blood for lab tests is not typically drawn from a peripheral catheter once the infusion has been initiated. In certain practice areas, such as emergency departments and pre-hospital care, blood samples may be taken after the vein has been accessed and prior to infusion of fluids. This reduces the number of needlesticks, thus lessening the amount of pain and the chance of infection.

Sometimes a patient's peripheral catheter is used only for intermittent infusions. In this case, an **injection cap,** or **PRN adaptor,** (see Figure 3-20 page 56) is inserted into the hub. This cap, also known as a lock, is made of self-healing latex so that a needle or, preferably, a needleless injection system can penetrate it when medications and/or fluids are to be administered. A peripheral catheter that is used for intermittent infusion needs to be flushed with a saline or heparin solution after every use or at least twice daily if not in use. A **saline flush** is an injection of saline solution to flush out, or clean, the catheter. A **heparin flush** is an injection of a diluted solution of the anticoagulant medication heparin into the catheter to prevent blood from clotting in it between uses. An intermittent IV that is capped and flushed on a regular basis is sometimes called either a saline lock or a heparin lock. The flushing process makes use of 2 mL to 5 mL of either normal saline solution (NSS) or dilute heparin. The solution to be used for flushing is determined by the physician's orders or by facility protocols. Health care facilities frequently stock prefilled syringes that can be attached to a needleless cannula. After the PRN adaptor is disinfected, the cannula is inserted and the tubing is unclamped. The flushing usually begins with a brief aspiration for blood return to evaluate patency of the system. The contents of the syringe are instilled, and continuous pressure is put on the plunger as the syringe is withdrawn and the tubing is reclamped. The cap is self-sealing, so it will not leak.

Steel Needle

The wing-tipped, or butterfly, catheter is the most commonly used steel needle (Figure 3-4). It is named after the wing-like plastic tabs at the base of the needle. Butterfly catheters are used to deliver small quantities of medicines, to deliver fluids via the scalp veins in infants, and sometimes to draw blood samples (although not routinely, because the small diameter may damage blood cells). Butterfly needles are shorter and have a smaller diameter (gauge), which makes them easier to insert into small or fragile veins.

Rigid needle devices such as the butterfly are used only occasionally for short-term administration. Because winged-tipped needles account for the majority of reported needlestick injuries in IV therapy, they are being phased out completely. OSHA safety guidelines recommend flexible catheters and needleless **cannula systems** to reduce the risk of accidental needlesticks. A cannula system is a venous access device in the form of a plastic tube; during insertion, its **lumen** (the open space in the center of the tube) is usually occupied by a **trocar** (needle). Once the tube is in place, the needle is removed and discarded.

Wing-tipped devices are now available with flexible over-the-needle catheters; the wings replace the hub for easier insertion. After the needle has been inserted, it can be withdrawn from the flexible catheter. This new system, which is equipped with a safety sheath to cover the needle as soon as it is withdrawn from the vein, meets OSHA safety standards.

Figure 3-4   This wing-tipped butterfly device has a safety sheath to prevent needlesticks during IV access.

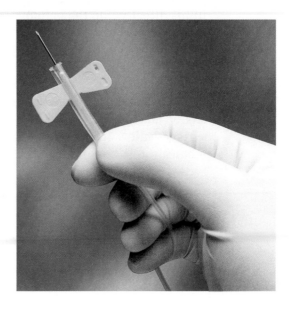

Figure 3-5 A needleless syringe is used to inject medication into an existing IV.

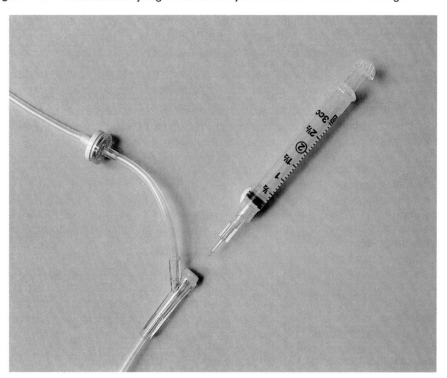

Needleless Systems

Although a needle is necessary to pierce the skin in order to start an IV, needleless systems can be used to add medications and secondary lines to an IV. These systems must comply with engineered sharps injury protection rules established by OSHA. As you learned in Chapter 2, these rules require that needles or other sharps devices be built with attributes—for example, devices to blunt, sheath, or withdraw the sharp—that effectively reduce the risk of exposure to blood-borne pathogens.

Needleless syringes are used to administer medication through already-established IV lines (Figure 3-5). These syringes can deliver medication and fluids directly into the patient's veins. Adding medication through existing lines has several advantages. First, the patient can receive IV medications quickly through the existing injection port without having to be punctured repeatedly. Second, because the syringes do not have needles, accidental needlesticks to patients and health care workers are avoided. Third, an IV system with a needleless syringe allows for more than one drug to be administered at a time, provided that the drugs are compatible. Fourth, needleless syringes allow for a drug to be delivered on a periodic basis and for the medication to be diluted.

Midline Peripheral Catheters and Peripherally Inserted Central Catheters

Any catheter placed between the antecubital area and the head of the clavicle is called a **midline catheter.** This type of catheter is inserted into the arm near the inside of the elbow and is threaded up inside the vein to a length of 6 inches (Figure 3-6). Because the end of the catheter reaches a much larger

Figure 3-6 A midline or a PICC catheter is inserted between the antecubital area and the head of the clavicle by using a shielded introducer like the one shown here.

Introducer assembly

(Before activation)

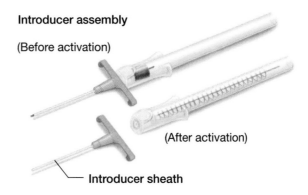

(After activation)

Introducer sheath

vein that has more blood flow, the midline catheter causes less irritation of the vein. This catheter can last about 6 weeks, which makes it a perfect catheter for a short course of antibiotics but not practical for long-term IV therapy.

Because the midline catheter is so soft and the end is well inside the vein, it is much less likely to become dislodged than is a peripheral IV. The insertion site will still need to be covered with a transparent dressing to keep it clean and dry. Because this catheter is near the elbow, the patient should wear a long-sleeved shirt to protect and hide it. The patient can do most normal activities with a midline catheter, except swimming, as long as he or she is careful with the arm.

As you learned in Chapter 1, a peripherally inserted central catheter (PICC) is inserted into a peripheral vein, usually in the arm, and then is carefully advanced upward until the catheter reaches the superior vena cava or the right atrium. The PICC catheter can have two parallel compartments, each with its own external connector (double lumen), or can have a single tube and connector (single lumen) (Figure 3-7). From the outside, a single-lumen PICC resembles a peripheral IV except that the tubing is slightly wider.

Figure 3-7 PICC and midline catheters are similar to peripheral catheters but are wider and may have two parallel compartments.

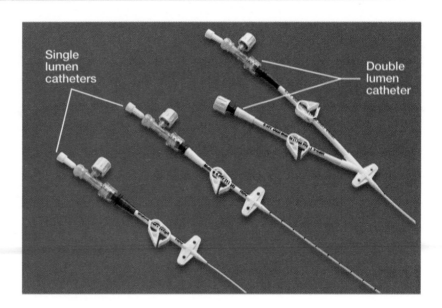

Single lumen catheters

Double lumen catheter

Central Venous Catheters

Catheters that take a more direct route into central veins are collectively known as **central venous lines.** These catheters are inserted by physicians or other specially trained personnel. The two types of central venous catheters are those that are permanently placed under the skin with no catheter coming out through the skin (internal catheters, or ports) and those that come out through the skin (external catheters).

The choice of an internal or external catheter usually depends on the specific needs and preferences of the patient and the health care provider. If the catheter is going to be used frequently and for infusions lasting several hours, an external catheter is preferable because it does not require a needle to be placed through the skin to deliver the needed medications. When internal catheters are accessed frequently, the skin overlying the reservoir will often become weak and the frequent puncturing may lead to infections. The external catheter requires a sterile dressing that should be changed once or twice a day and may need to be periodically flushed with heparin, as discussed earlier in this chapter, to prevent it from clotting. The internal catheter, because it is completely under the skin, requires no special care when it is not being accessed. From the patient's perspective, an internal catheter is preferable, but it may not be an option if the patient's catheter requires frequent or continuous use.

Centrally Placed External Catheters

One brand of centrally placed external catheter is the Groshong catheter. The Groshong catheter has a valve at the tip that prevents blood from backing up into the catheter, so heparin is not necessary. Groshong catheters are usually thinner and more flexible than other types of catheters, and they do not require the bulky clamp that other catheters have. After the catheter is inserted, a chest x-ray is required to make sure the tip is in the right location above the heart. The insertion site is covered with a transparent dressing that must be kept clean and dry at all times; it is changed and the site is cleaned once a week or more often (Figure 3-8). Groshong catheters usually last for

Figure 3-8 A Groshong catheter is centrally placed directly above the heart and is usually left in place for 6 weeks to 6 months. A weekly cleaning of the site is usually done.

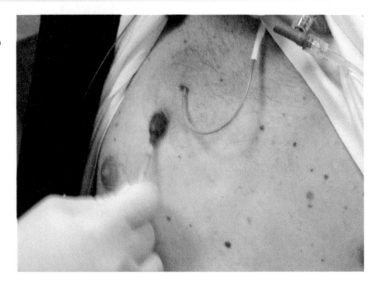

Figure 3-9 A Hickman catheter is a centrally placed catheter that is tunneled under the skin which reduces the risk of infection from the skin surface.

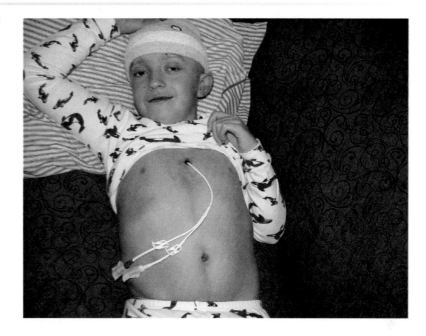

6 weeks to 6 months, although they have been known to last even longer. Blood can be drawn from a Groshong catheter, which replaces the need for venipuncture each time lab tests are required. The Groshong requires a saline flush after each use or once daily if not in use.

Another type of central line, called a Hickman or Broviac catheter, is inserted into the target vein and then "tunneled" under the skin to emerge a short distance away (Figure 3-9). This method reduces the risk of infection, because bacteria from the skin surface are not able to travel directly into the vein; also, these catheters are made of materials that resist infection and clotting. A Dacron cuff on the catheter just inside the skin tunnel forms a seal with the patient's skin that prevents bacteria from entering the bloodstream. These tunneled catheters are usually more comfortable than other external catheters for patients to "wear."

The tunneled catheter is surgically inserted during an outpatient procedure in which the patient is under local anesthesia. The catheter exit is usually near the nipple area, but patients should discuss the exit site with their physician prior to insertion; patients who always sleep on their right side, for example, might prefer to have the catheter exit on the left. Physicians will try to accommodate patients' requests but will need to choose a placement that works best with each patient's veins and chest.

After the insertion surgery, most patients find that the shoulder area is somewhat sore for a few days but that the pain is tolerable. Once home, the patient (or a family member) must clean the catheter exit site and change the gauze dressing daily. For the first two weeks, the gauze dressing must remain dry and intact at all times; the patient should cover the site with a transparent dressing or with plastic wrap while taking a shower or should take a tub bath while keeping the chest dry. After two weeks, if the dressing gets wet in the shower or tub, the patient can change it immediately afterward. Once the exit site has healed completely (usually in 6 to 8 weeks), the patient can just clean the area with a bit of soap and water and then pat it dry and cover it with a plain bandage. During the day, the external catheter should be taped to the patient's chest so that it does not dangle or catch on something. The catheter is usually not noticeable under T-shirts or even tank tops. Once the shoulder is no longer sore, the patient is able to resume all normal daily activities except swimming. Some doctors will allow their patients to swim in a clean pool if the catheter site is fully healed and is covered with a transparent occlusion dressing meant to keep out water. Swimming in rivers, lakes, or oceans is usually not allowed, and some doctors do not allow their patients to swim or use hot tubs at all because of possible contamination or exposure to pathogens.

The Broviac catheter requires a saline flush after each medication or every 1 to 7 days if not in use. The Hickman catheter requires a saline and heparin flush after every medication or at least once daily if not in use. With the physician's consent, blood can be drawn from a tunneled catheter. Tunneled catheters are designed to be permanent. In the event that the physician decides to remove the catheter, the process is relatively easy and painless. The patient may feel a slight stinging sensation when the catheter is pulled out.

Centrally Placed Internal Ports

A port (often referred to by brand names such as Port-a-Cath or MediPort) is a central venous line that does not have an external connector; instead, it has a reservoir implanted under the skin, usually in the chest area (Figure 3-10). The small titanium reservoir has a rubber stopper that is attached to the catheter entering the subclavian vein. The reservoir and the catheter are surgically implanted during an outpatient procedure in which the patient is under local anesthesia and IV sedation. These catheters are usually not noticeable under the skin but may sometimes show as a small lump. To access a port, the health care worker first locates and cleans the site and then inserts a special needle through the skin and into the rubber stopper. This procedure can be implemented for each dose of medication, or the needle can be left in place, covered with a plastic dressing, and changed weekly. Ports cause little inconvenience and have a low risk of infection; they are commonly used for patients on long-term intermittent treatment such as chemotherapy.

Because of the procedures required to access the port, these catheters are not recommended for patients who need daily or more frequent medications. Internal ports are perfect for a patient who receives medication on an

Figure 3-10 A Port-A-Cath is one type of centrally placed port. It is implanted under the skin for long-term intermittent IV therapy such as chemotherapy.

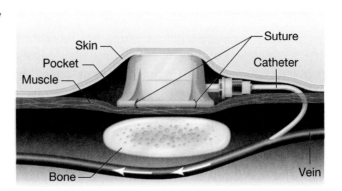

intermittent schedule, such as once a week or one full week every six weeks. Ports are made to withstand 2000 needle entries. Most patients develop a callus by the insertion site that prevents pain when the needle is placed through the skin. Patients can be taught to clean the site and self-access the port with a needle, but the procedure is difficult to learn and complicated to do. Another type of implanted port is placed in the arm near the elbow, and the catheter line is threaded up the vein to the superior vena cava, but this arm port offers no particular advantage over a chest port, and it tends to have more complications and is harder for the patient to self-access because two hands are required for the procedure.

When a port is not accessed, it is hardly visible and requires no care other than a once-monthly flushing with heparin. Patients with unaccessed ports can swim, though sometimes a doctor will recommend that the site be covered with a waterproof plastic dressing. Because the skin is an excellent barrier to bacteria, unaccessed ports rarely become infected. However, if a port is accessed frequently or if the needle access is left in place for extended periods, the odds of infection become greater for a port than for a tunneled catheter. With a physician's consent, blood for lab tests can be drawn from a port.

Patient Education & Communication

Long Term IV Therapy

Patients who will be receiving long-term IV therapy must be provided with information on how to care for the IV site. Each patient should be taught the basics of IV site care, be given written information about caring for the site, be allowed to ask questions, taught the signs of problems and contact information in case a problem occurs.

Checkpoint Question 3-2

1. Which is the most common type of peripheral IV access device? Why?

   _____

   _____

 Before you continue to the next section, answer the previous Checkpoint Question and complete the Catheters and Access Devices activity under Chapter 3 on the student CD.

3-3 Venous Access Device Selection

The size and type of venous access device (catheter) is usually chosen for a patient by the health care practitioner who will be starting the IV therapy. You should become familiar with the selection process in order to develop your competency in providing IV therapy.

Factors to Consider

To select the proper catheter for a patient, the health care practitioner must consider five factors:

1. The type of fluids to be administered
   - Will the patient also receive IV medication?
   - Will the patient possibly need blood or blood products?
2. The length of time that the patient is expected to be receiving IV fluids
   - Will the infusion be continuous or intermittent?
3. The location, size, and condition of the patient's veins
4. The patient's age, level of activity, and consciousness
   - Is there a danger that the patient will disturb the infusion site?
5. The method used to control the infusion rate
   - Will the infusion rate be controlled with a pump?
   - Will the infusion rate be controlled by gravity?

Catheter Sizes

Catheters (and needles) are sized by their length and diameter. The lengths vary from ½ inch to 2 inches. The diameter is called the *gauge*; the smaller the diameter, the larger the gauge. Catheters and their introducer needle come in sizes that range from 14 to 26 gauge. Therefore, a 22-gauge catheter is smaller than a 14-gauge catheter. Obviously, a catheter with a larger diameter can deliver more fluid. To deliver large amounts of fluid, the health care practitioner would select a large vein and use a 14-gauge or 16-gauge catheter. To administer medications, the practitioner can use an 18-gauge or 20-gauge catheter in a smaller vein.

The largest catheter is the 14-gauge catheter, and it is normally reserved for trauma situations or for surgery. This size allows rapid delivery of fluids; if a patient is hemorrhaging, for example, a 14-gauge catheter is necessary to administer blood products, including packed cells. The most commonly used catheter sizes are 18 and 20 gauge. Most adult patients have veins that can accommodate catheters this size, and the diameter is adequate for the infusion of fluids as well as blood. The smaller access devices, such as 22-gauge to 26-gauge catheters, are used for elderly patients, for infants and young children, and for patients who are dehydrated or who have small or poorly accessible veins.

The health care practitioner will always select the shortest and smallest cannula sufficient to deliver the prescribed fluids, blood products, and medication (Figure 3-11). A catheter that is too large can hamper adequate blood flow around the catheter and can lead to phlebitis. Longer and larger

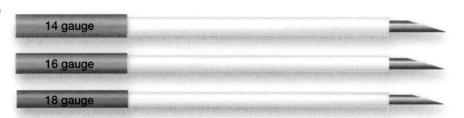

Figure 3-11 The gauge of the needle relates to the diameter: the larger the number, the narrower the needle diameter.

14 gauge

16 gauge

18 gauge

catheters increase the risk to the patient of thrombus formation, infection, or infiltration. Additionally a large catheter can make starting an IV more difficult and cause the patient unnecessary pain.

Checkpoint Questions 3-3

1. What factors do you need to consider when choosing the size and type of venous access device?

_____

_____

2. How would you determine whether to use a 24-gauge or an 18-gauge needle for a peripheral IV?

_____

_____

Before you continue to the next section, answer the previous Checkpoint Questions and complete the Venous Access Device Selection activity under Chapter 3 on the student CD.

3-4 Administration Equipment

A standard IV administration set, also called a **primary administration set,** is attached to a prefilled sterile bag of fluid and consists of a drip chamber, a long sterile tube with a clamp to regulate or stop the flow, a connector that attaches to the access device, and connectors for attaching another infusion

Figure 3-12 A primary administration line includes a drip chamber, a long sterile tube, connectors, and a clamp to regulate the flow of the infusion.

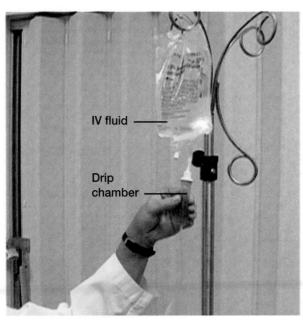

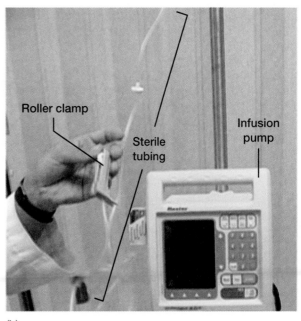

(a)   (b)

set on the same line (Figure 3-12). The drip chamber allows the fluid to flow one drop at a time, which reduces air bubbles and makes it easy for you to observe the flow rate. A **secondary administration set** is used for adding a medication to a continuous fluid drip. Other devices used during administration include filters, extension sets, adaptors, and connectors.

Primary Administration Sets

The tubing of a primary administration set is connected directly to the IV site and to the fluid that is to be infused. The tubing should be long enough for the patient to move around but should not touch the floor. The primary administration set must be compatible with the infusion pump to be used. (Infusion pumps, discussed in the section titled IV Regulators, are electronic devices that control the rate of an IV infusion.) The infusion rates of primary administration sets are calibrated by the manufacturer, and the drip rate is printed on the package and sometimes even on the administration set itself.

Administration sets come in two sizes: macrodrip and microdrip (Figure 3-13). Macrodrip tubing allows larger drops—10 to 20 drops per **milliliter (mL)**—to form and fall into the drip chamber. (A milliliter is a unit of measure in the metric system; the volume of fluid infused during IV therapy is measured in milliliters.) Macrodrip tubing is used for infusions of 80 mL/hour or more and is always used for operating room infusions. Microdrip tubing allows smaller drops (60 drops/mL) to enter the drip chamber. Microdrip tubing is used for infusions of less than 80 mL/hour and is often used for slower infusions, such as KVO infusions. (*KVO* means "keep vein open"; a KVO infusion is a very slow rate that is just enough to keep the vein open in case of emergency or if medications need to be administered.) Microdrip tubing is especially useful for pediatric and critical-care IVs, when very small volumes are used and accuracy is extremely important. Accidental increases in volume can be fatal in these situations.

Flow rate information is important if infusion is to be delivered by gravity flow. Unless you are using an electronic pump to deliver the fluid at precise amounts, you will need to know how to set a flow rate yourself. Flow rate is usually determined by counting the number of drops that fall into the drip chamber in one minute. To set flow rate accurately, you must

Figure 3-13 Microdrip tubing allows for 60 drops of fluid in every one milliliter. Macrodrip tubing allows for larger drops.

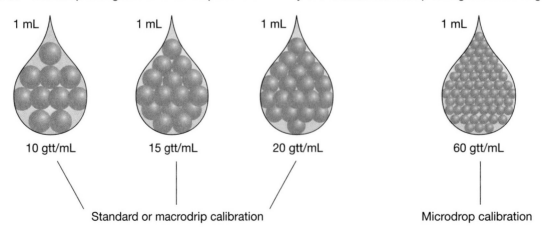

1 mL — 10 gtt/mL   1 mL — 15 gtt/mL   1 mL — 20 gtt/mL   1 mL — 60 gtt/mL

Standard or macrodrip calibration   Microdrop calibration

Figure 3-14 Roller and slide clamps control the flow rate of an IV but should remain open when the fluid is connected to an electronic infusion device.

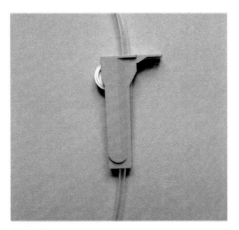

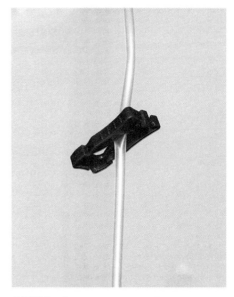

(a) Roller clamp.

(b) Slide clamp.

know what size administration set you are using (microdrip or macrodrip). For complete instructions on flow rate calculations and practice problems, see Chapter 8.

To measure the flow rate, squeeze and release the drip chamber until it is half filled with IV solution. Having fluid in the drip chamber makes it easier for you to count the drops that fall into it from the bag. Use roller or screw clamps to set or adjust the flow rate of the IV solution (Figure 3-14). A slide clamp is used to shut off the IV solution's flow completely without disturbing the flow rate setting. Some infusion sets are equipped with a "dial-a-flow" controller that can be set to the prescribed milliliter rate per hour (Figure 3-15). The primary administration set may also include an injection port that allows you to inject medications or compatible fluids into the primary line or to attach a second IV line. The IV bags themselves may also have ports that allow additives to be injected directly into the solution.

Figure 3-15 The infusion set is equipped with a dial-a-flow controller that can be preset to deliver a prescribed rate of infusion in milliliters per hour.

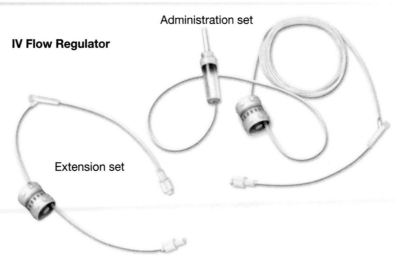

Administration set

IV Flow Regulator

Extension set

Primary tubes are available in various lengths. When choosing the length of tubing, consider the patient's mobility status. Longer tubing, for example, permits a patient to move from the bed to a bedside chair or commode without having to move the IV pole or pump. Do not use a tube that is long enough to dangle on the floor. A catheter can be dislodged if its tubing is stepped on or has furniture rolled over it. Contact with the floor can also cause contamination.

Secondary Administration Sets

A secondary administration set, used for intermittent infusions or IV push medications, allows you to access the patient's vein without moving the catheter or causing trauma to the IV site. The secondary injection port is covered with a plastic cap that can be penetrated with a needle, with a needleless syringe cannula, or with secondary tubing that has a needleless access cannula. The port cap can be penetrated numerous times without leaking because it has self-sealing properties.

A secondary administration set may also require extension tubing, a piggyback set, or Y tubing. Each of these items has a specific purpose, but all three items are considered secondary tubing. Short **extension tubing** provides easy access for intermittent infusions and also adds length to the primary set when necessary (Figure 3-16).

A piggyback, or secondary, set is used to administer IV medications such as antibiotics through an existing IV access. The piggyback set consists of a connector, a long tube, and a container of medication. A needleless device is used to attach the piggyback connector to the primary injection port, which must be cleaned prior to access. The medication bag usually contains 50 to 100 mL of fluid in addition to the medication.

Figure 3-16 An extension tube with a needleless system provides a location for intermittent infusions or IV push medications. Circled in these figures are the injection ports available for needless injections.

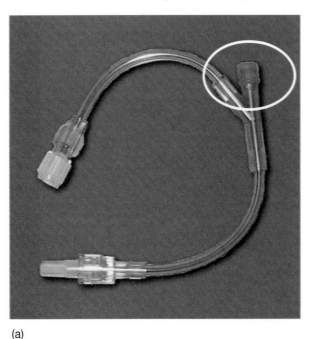 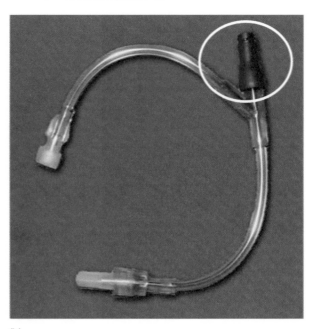

(a)   (b)

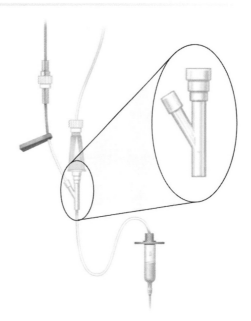

Figure 3-17 The Y connector is used for blood administration or multiple infusions into one IV site.

A **Y set** or a Y set with micro filters is used for blood administration. The Y set has two short arms of IV tubing, each with a spike; these arms come together at the drip chamber. Below the drip chamber is an inline micro-aggregate filter. The blood bag is attached to one arm, and the other arm is for 0.9% saline, which is used to prime the tubing before the infusion is started. Other IV fluids are not used with blood transfusions; dextrose, for example, can cause cellular changes in the blood (Figure 3-17).

Accessory Devices for IV Administration

Filters prevent impurities and particulate matter from entering the blood-stream of the patient (Figure 3-18). Filters may be built into an infusion set or are sometimes added to the administration set. In general, added filters

Figure 3-18 Filters, frequently part of an IV administration set, prevent impurities and particulate matter from entering the bloodstream.

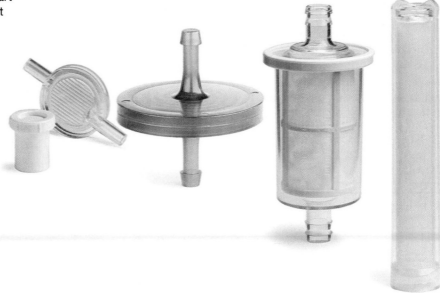

Figure 3-19 Stopcocks allow more than one fluid to flow into the patient through the same IV site. Pictured here is a 3-way stopcock.

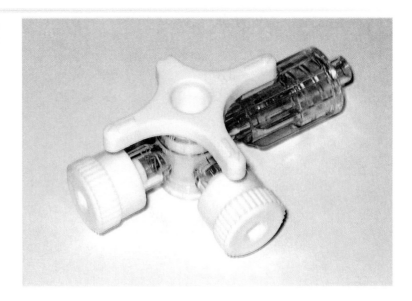

are not recommended, but when they are used, the manufacturer's directions must be followed precisely.

Connecters and adaptors may already be in place or may be added to an IV set. A **stopcock** device controls the direction of flow of the IV fluid (Figure 3-19). Stopcocks allow more than one fluid to flow into the patient through the same IV site. Stopcocks can be three-way or four-way. A three-way stopcock allows two different fluids to flow into the patient at separate times. A four-way stopcock allows two separate fluids to flow into the patient at the same time or at separate times. T ports, J loops, and U connectors are used to temporarily disconnect a patient from a continuous IV. These connectors make it convenient for patients to get out of bed, to walk, or to take a shower.

As you learned in the section titled Over-the-Needle Catheter, a PRN adaptor, or injection cap, is used for intermittent IV therapy. The PRN adaptor is placed on an IV site when continuous therapy is no longer needed but intermittent access is. This adaptor has an injection site that allows for needleless access when medication or fluids must be administered (Figure 3-20). PRN adaptors are flushed on a regular basis with saline or heparin to ensure that the IV catheter stays patent (open).

Figure 3-20 A PRN ("as needed") adaptor is placed on the end of an IV site when IV access is needed only intermittently.

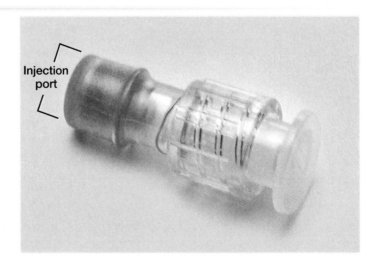

Injection port

An IV pole is another accessory device for IV infusion. These poles are used alone or with an electronic infusion pump. IV poles are typically on wheels for easy movement. Some IV poles are attached directly to the bed or stretcher.

Safety and Infection Control

Maintain a Closed IV System

An IV that is attached to a patient and in progress is called a closed system. When an IV line is breeched (opened)—to add accessory devices, for example—it creates an entry port for infection. Ideally, you should add accessory devices such as filters, stopcocks, connectors, and adaptors to the IV system before you connect the IV to the patient. If you must add accessory devices after the infusion has begun, use strict aseptic technique to prevent contamination of the system.

Checkpoint Questions 3-4

1. What are the differences between a macrodrip administration set and a microdrip one?

_____

_____

2. When should a secondary administration set be used?

_____

_____

Before you continue to the next section, answer the previous Checkpoint Questions and complete the Administration Equipment activity under Chapter 3 on the student CD.

3-5 Fluids

Most IV fluids come in soft, flexible plastic containers, although glass containers may be used for certain medications (Figures 3-21 and 3-22). IV fluid bags can hold solution amounts that range from 50 mL to 2000 mL, but they most often contain 500 or 1000 mL of solution. Smaller bags of fluid (50 to 250 mL) are usually used for IV medications (Figure 3-23). All IV bags are labeled with their contents by the manufacturer. Some IV bags include an injection port so that additional medication can be added to the solution. The amount of fluid that a patient receives is considered part of that patient's intake and must be recorded. When you are infusing IV fluid into a patient, you will follow specific guidelines for monitoring and recording this information at regular intervals. See Chapters 6 and 7 for more information about monitoring and documenting IV fluid intake.

Plastic IV fluid bags are sometimes covered with a transparent plastic wrap that must be removed before administration. If the pharmacist has added medication to the solution, the plastic wrap may already be removed. In either case, check the IV fluid bag for leaks or punctures. Also, check the

Figure 3-21 Most IV fluids come in soft, flexible containers such as this one.

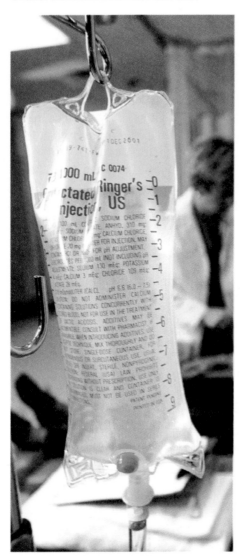

Figure 3-22 Occasionally, certain medications must be prepared in and administered from a glass bottle.

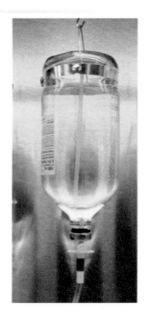

Figure 3-23 The ADD-Vantage system provides the labeled medication and the fluid it is to be mixed with when infused.

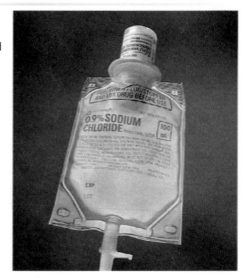

fluid for clarity. Do not use bags that are damaged or contain fluids that appear cloudy or have particles. Make a note of the type of fluid and the lot number, and notify the pharmacy or central storage so that the entire supply of IV fluids can be checked and discarded if necessary.

Safety and Infection Control

Check and Label the IV Bag Properly

In addition to checking the IV fluid bag for damage and checking the fluid for clarity, always check the bag contents and the expiration date printed on the label. For safety reasons, never mark directly on an IV bag; it may cause damage, seep through to the contents of the bag, or simply not be legible. Look for a printed label already affixed to the bag, or attach a new sticky label.

Checkpoint Question 3-5

1. How should plastic IV fluid bags be marked?

_____

_____

Before you continue to the next section, answer the previous Checkpoint Question and complete the Fluids activity under Chapter 3 on the student CD.

3-6 IV Regulators

IVs must be monitored and regulated to ensure that the proper type of fluid enters the body at the correct rate. IVs are monitored either manually or electronically. Electronic IV regulators, collectively known as **electronic flow control devices,** include infusion pumps, rate controllers, syringe pumps, and patient-controlled analgesia pumps. In order to properly maintain and monitor an IV, you must have an understanding of both manual monitoring and monitoring regulated by electronic flow control devices.

Manual Monitoring

When electronic devices are not feasible or available, IVs are monitored and regulated manually (Figure 3-24). Manual regulation of an IV is done infrequently; however, you must be familiar with manual regulation in case an electronic pump or electrical power to run a pump is not available. For an IV with using *gravity drip*, hang the bag about 36 inches above the level of the patient and use the clamp to regulate the rate. If the patient requires a high flow rate and the IV access device is large enough to accommodate it, you can place an inflatable cuff around the IV bag to force the fluid into the patient. Gravity infusion is affected by many factors, which are described in Table 3-1. Chapter 6 provides more information about IV monitoring.

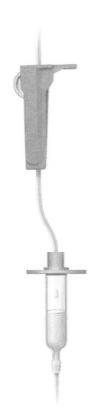

Figure 3-24 A gravity drip IV is usually regulated by a roller clamp such as this one. The number of drops per minute is counted in the drip chamber.

TABLE 3-1 Variables that Affect Gravity Infusion

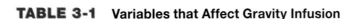

Condition	Effect on Rate of Infusion
Temperature of fluids	Cold fluids drip slower than warm fluids.
Height of container	The higher the container is above the site, the faster the fluids will flow.
Position of drip chamber	If the drip chamber is tilted, the drops will be larger.
Coughing	Coughing can slow the flow rate temporarily.
Increased blood pressure	An increase in blood pressure can slow the flow rate temporarily.
Length of catheter	A shorter catheter causes a faster flow. A longer catheter causes a resistance that slows the flow.

Careful IV Monitoring is Always Required

Manual control of IVs is not recommended because the variables make regulation difficult and unpredictable. Use of an electronic flow control device, however, does not replace the need for careful monitoring. Always monitor IV infusions at regular intervals and whenever you enter the patient's room.

Infusion Pumps

An **infusion pump** allows precise control over an IV's flow rate and the total amount of fluid delivered (Figure 3-25). The infusion pump is the most predictable infusion method because it does not rely on gravity; instead, it forces the IV solution through the tubing. The pump on this infusion device applies pressure sufficient to deliver a set volume of liquid every minute into the patient's vein; the desired flow rate can be set either in mL/hour or by dosage. A sensor on the infusion pump sounds an alarm if the flow rate cannot be maintained or if the bag is empty. When you encounter a slow flow rate, look for a blockage or other resistance in the vein, for a kink in the tubing, or for a catheter that has dislodged. Sometimes the equipment will continue to pump IV fluid even though the catheter is out of the vein. You must monitor the patient regularly for signs that the IV fluid is improperly entering the tissue outside the vein, a situation known as *infiltration*. Infiltration is indicated by swelling, coolness, or discomfort at the insertion site; it is discussed in more detail in Chapter 6. Infusion pumps are used to regulate

Figure 3-25 Infusion pumps apply pressure to deliver a set volume of liquid every minute.

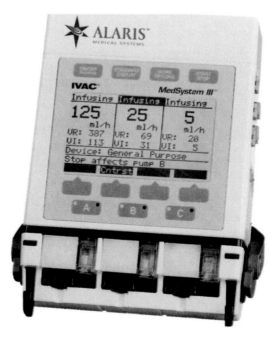

peripheral as well as central vein infusions. However, an infusion pump should always be used in central veins because of their higher pressure.

Rate Controllers

A **rate controller** relies on gravity to infuse an IV solution, but no clamp is used to adjust the flow rate. Instead, tubing is threaded through the controller, where a pincher maintains a preset flow rate. The controller is attached to a sensor that measures the number of drops or the volume of solution that is delivered. An alarm sounds when the preset flow rate cannot be maintained. Rate controllers do not actually pump the fluid; they just monitor its rate of delivery.

Figure 3-26   A syringe pump provides precise control over delivery of IV medications.

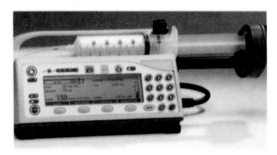

Syringe Pumps

A **syringe pump** allows a syringe to be inserted into the pump unit (Figure 3-26). The syringe can deliver medication or fluids that cannot be combined with other medications or solutions. Syringe pumps are useful for pediatric medications as well as for medications that must be administered at a precisely controlled rate. Syringe pumps are often used when a medication must be administered within a half hour or less, but they are also used for longer time periods. One common use of the syringe pump is for pregnant women during delivery. The physician may induce the woman's labor by using a syringe pump to administer oxytocin, a medication that causes uterine contractions.

Patient-Controlled Analgesia Pumps

Patients in pain, including pain from cancer or surgery, use **patient-controlled analgesia (PCA) pumps** or devices to administer their own pain medication (Figure 3-27). The PCA pump allows patients to control their own medication—within limits preset according to the physician's order—by pressing a button on a handheld device. The PCA pump helps monitor the effectiveness of the pain relief prescription by recording the number of times the patient presses the button. This device provides the patient with quick access to pain medication but does not allow the patient to receive more than the prescribed amount of medication.

Figure 3-27 A patient-controlled analgesia (PCA) pump gives the patient limited control over the amount of medication administered.

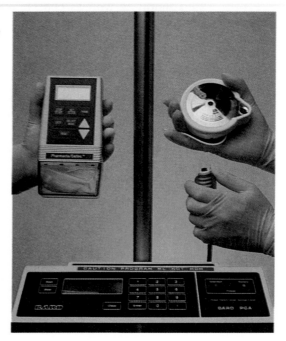

Patient Controlled Analgesia

When your patient is given a PCA pump for pain medication, you must teach the patient how to use the device properly. Your instructions to the patient should include the following points:

- *How to work the PCA pump.* Explain to the patient that pain medication is administered when the button is pushed. Make sure the patient understands that a prescribed delay time between doses ensures that the patient cannot overdose on the medication.
- *How to use the button.* Demonstrate use of the button on the hand-held device, and place the device within reach of the patient. Put the device in the patient's hand if necessary.
- *How to determine need.* Instruct the patient to avoid severe pain by administering frequent small doses as soon as pain occurs.
- *How to assess pain.* Ask the patient to rate the level of pain on a scale of 1 to 10. Explain to the patient that this information is used to determine whether the medication is successfully controlling the pain.

You will also need to instruct the patient's family not to initiate medication doses for the patient.

Volume-Control Sets

Volume-control sets (some brand names are Buretrol, Soluset, and Volutrol) are used with manual IV setups and electronic rate controllers to improve the accuracy of fluid infusion, especially for small volumes of medication or fluid (Figure 3-28). Volume-control sets are calibrated in 1 milliliter increments, and their total volume capacity ranges from 100 to 150 mL. The

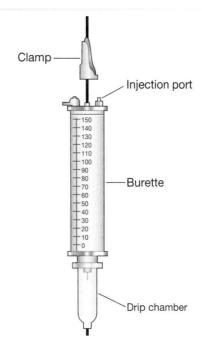

Figure 3-28 Volume-control sets allow small volumes of medications or fluids to be administered and monitored frequently.

Clamp

Injection port

150
140
130
120
110
100
90
80
70
60
50
40
30
20
10
0

Burette

Drip chamber

medication is introduced through an injection port into a burette—a chamber designed to hold a smaller, controlled amount of fluid. An exact amount of IV fluid is added as diluent to the burette chamber, where the medication and IV fluid are mixed. The solution is delivered to the patient in microdrips. Volume-control sets are often used in critical-care or pediatric IVs, where small doses of medication and fluid must be administered.

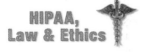

HIPAA, Law & Ethics

Troubleshoot the Infusion Pump

Electronic infusion pumps are equipped with an alarm system to alert the health care staff of possible malfunctions. Although alarms that are continuously activated can be annoying to patients and staff, they should never be silenced for convenience. Your correct course of action is to troubleshoot the functioning of the pump and correct the problem; any other action would be considered negligent. A negligent act can lead to a malpractice suit, but more importantly, it may cause harm to the patient.

Troubleshooting

PCA Pump Instruction

You check on a patient who has just come out of surgery and is connected to a PCA pump. The handheld button is laying on the patient's bed. When you ask her to rate her pain, she says, "It is a 10. Can't you give me some medication so I don't hurt so much?"

What should you do?

_____

_____

Checkpoint Questions 3-6

1. What is a gravity drip?

_____

_____

2. How do infusion pumps control the flow of IV fluids?

_____

_____

3. How do syringe pumps differ from the pumps used to administer patient-controlled analgesics?

_____

_____

 Before you continue to the chapter summary, answer the previous Checkpoint Questions and complete the IV Regulators activity under Chapter 3 on the student CD.

Chapter Summary

- The most commonly used access device for peripheral IVs is the over-the-needle catheter. Used less frequently are the needle and syringe system and the steel needle.

- Midline peripheral catheters, peripherally inserted central catheters, and central IV lines come in various types and are designed to deliver fluids, nutrition, and medication over an extended period of time.

- Factors to be considered in the selection of a venous access device are the type of fluids to be administered; the length of time that the patient is expected to be receiving IV fluids; the location, size, and condition of the patient's veins; the age, level of activity, and consciousness of the patient; and the method used to control the infusion rate.

- Catheters and needles are sized by their diameter; this measurement is called the *gauge*. The gauge of access devices ranges from 14 to 26. The lower the number, the larger the diameter.

- Administration sets are either microdrip or macrodrip. The classification is determined by the size of the drop or the number of drops in a milliliter of fluid.

- The primary administration set is the main IV line; it consists of a drip chamber, sterile tube with a clamp, and connectors for the access device and other infusion sets. Secondary tubing can be extension sets to add length, Y sets for blood administration, and secondary administration sets that are used to infuse additional fluids or medications to the primary administration set.

- IV fluids are most commonly supplied in clear flexible plastic containers that must be labeled. However, the fluid bags should never be written on directly.

- Although IV infusions can be controlled and monitored manually, the most reliable method of control is an infusion pump. PCA pumps allow patients to control their own medication within prescribed limits. Syringe pumps allows for controlled administration of IV medications. Volume-control sets are used for accurate control of the amount of IV fluids that a patient receives.

Multiple Choice

1. Which of the following statements is true of the needle in an over-the-needle catheter?
   a. The needle is outside the catheter.
   b. The needle is used less frequently than a butterfly needle is.
   c. The needle is inside the catheter.
   d. The needle is left in place after insertion.

2. A microdrip administration set delivers more drops per milliliter because
   a. the fluid is warmer and higher.
   b. the roller clamp adjusts to allow fluid to move through the tubing faster.
   c. the venous access device has a larger diameter.
   d. a needle in the drip chamber controls the size of the drops.

3. The physician has ordered a blood transfusion for your patient. In addition to the unit of blood, what other equipment from this list will you need?
   1. 500 mL normal saline solution
   2. Y-tube administration device
   3. 1000 mL of D5W (5% dextrose in water)
   4. 26-gauge venous access device
   5. 18-gauge venous access device
   a. 2, 3, and 4
   b. 2 only
   c. 1, 2, and 5
   d. all of the above

4. Which of the following is the major advantage of an internal IV port?
   a. No flushing is required.
   b. An internal port carries less risk of infection.
   c. An internal port offers painless accessibility.
   d. A nurse can insert an internal port.

5. How is the midline catheter different from the peripherally inserted central catheter?
   a. The midline catheter can be inserted by a nurse.
   b. The midline catheter tip is placed between the antecubital space and the shoulder.
   c. The midline catheter can be concealed by a T-shirt or tank top.
   d. The two are the same; there is no difference.

Fill-in-the-Blank

6. The difference between a controller and a pump is that the _____ delivers a preselected volume by adding pressure to the system when needed.

7. The temperature of IV fluids can affect the rate of infusion because warm fluids drip _____ than cold fluids do.

8. Coughing and increased _____ can slow the rate of a gravity infusion.

9. The majority of reported needlesticks in IV therapy are related to the use of _____ needles.

10. The smaller the gauge number of the needle, the _____ the diameter.

Matching

Match the IV equipment with its description.

Equipment

_____ 11. Y set

_____ 12. microdrip administration set

_____ 13. PRN adaptor

_____ 14. PCA

_____ 15. Port-a-Cath

_____ 16. Angiocath

_____ 17. macrodrip administration set

_____ 18. stopcock

_____ 19. Buretrol

_____ 20. Broviac catheter

Description

a. an externally placed central catheter

b. commonly used to administer blood

c. an internally placed central catheter

d. delivers 10 to 20 drops per milliliter

e. delivers 60 drops per milliliter

f. also known as an injection cap

g. allows for more than one fluid to flow into an IV access device

h. one type of volume-control set

i. patient-controlled analgesia

j. a common over-the-needle catheter

Identification

Match the following supplies and equipment with the correct picture.

_____ **21.** infusion pump

_____ **22.** Angiocath

_____ **23.** PCA pump

_____ **24.** syringe pump

_____ **25.** PICC catheter

_____ **26.** PRN adaptor

_____ **27.** Y set

_____ **28.** needleless syringe

_____ **29.** Port-a-Cath

_____ **30.** wing-tipped butterfly

a.

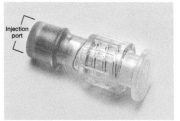

b.

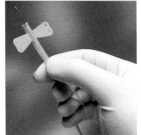

c.

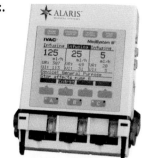

d.

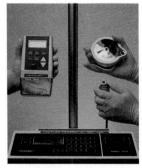

e.

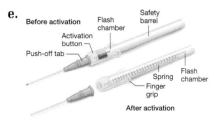

f.

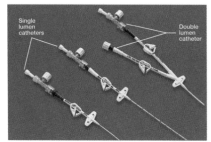

g.

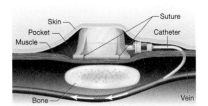

h.

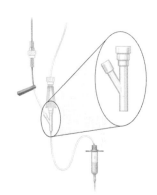

i.

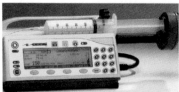

j.

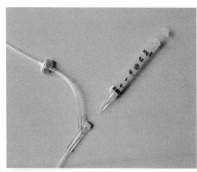

True/False

T   F   **31.** Peripheral access devices can be capped for intermittent IV therapy.

T   F   **32.** The simplest central venous access is into the subclavian vein.

T   F   **33.** Blood is considered a intravenous fluid.

T   F   **34.** Implantable ports have a higher incidence of infection than PICC lines do.

T   F   **35.** Central venous catheters are usually inserted by a physician.

What Should You Do? (Critical Thinking/Application Questions)

1. The report you just received about your patient states that her IV infusion is 1000 mL every 12 hours and that a new bag was added 2 hours ago. When you enter her room, you check the pump and find that the reading is appropriate for the amount ordered but that the fluid bag is only about half full. What would be your first action?

_____

_____

_____

Get Connected

Visit the McGraw-Hill Higher Education website for *Intravenous Therapy for Health Care Personnel* at **www.mhhe.com/healthcareskills** to complete the following activities.

1. In the ever-changing health care field, it is critical that the demand for continuing education be fulfilled. LITE (League of Intravenous Therapy Education) is a national educational association for infusion therapy, vascular access, home care, oncology, acute care, and extended care. In addition to offering educational seminars for health care professionals, support personnel, and students, LITE works to establish guidelines that promote safe, efficient, and cost-effective intravenous therapy in a multitude of care settings. Visit their website at **http://www.lite.org** and find an educational seminar you would like to attend.

2. Journal articles provide up-to-date information on changes, improvements, and alerts about procedures and equipment. The Internet is a good source for journal articles because many journals now have e-copies of articles as well as e-copy subscriptions available. Search the Internet, find a journal on IV therapy, and obtain an e-copy.

Using the Student CD

Now that you have completed the material in Chapter 3, return to the student CD and complete any chapter activities you have not yet done. Practice your terminology with the Key Term Concentration game. Review the chapter material with the Spin the Wheel game. Take the final chapter test, complete the troubleshooting question, and e-mail or print your results to document your proficiency for this chapter.

Intravenous Fluids, Components, and Compatibility

4

Chapter Outline

I. Introduction

II. Types and Uses of IV Fluids
   a. Sodium Chloride Solutions
   b. Dextrose Solutions
   c. Solutions with a Combination of Sodium Chloride and Dextrose
   d. Multiple Electrolyte Solutions
   e. Plasma Expanders
   f. Blood and Blood Products
      i. ABO Blood Groups
      ii. Rh Factor
      iii. Blood Transfusions

III. Additives
   a. Parenteral Nutrition
   b. Heparin
   c. Insulin
   d. Electrolytes and Vitamins

IV. Compatibility

V. Common IV Medications
   a. Classification of Medications
      i. Anti-infectives
      ii. Cardiovascular Medications
      iii. Central Nervous System Medications
      iv. Gastrointestinal Medications
      v. Chemotherapeutic Agents
   b. Administration of IV Medications

Learning Outcomes

- Differentiate among hypotonic, isotonic, and hypertonic fluids.
- Describe the uses for solutions containing sodium chloride, dextrose, a combination of sodium chloride and dextrose, and electrolytes.
- Discuss the purpose for infusing blood or blood products.
- Relate the importance of ABO and Rh compatibility to the infusion of blood or blood products.

- Describe the purpose of parenteral nutrition.
- List factors that affect compatibility of IV solutions and medications.
- Describe your responsibilities in avoiding incompatibility problems.
- Compare the advantages and disadvantages of IV medication administration.
- Identify the different classes of IV medications.
- Describe your responsibility in the safe administration of IV medications.

Key Terms

ABO system	incompatibility
anaphylaxis	isotonic solutions
blood component	maintenance fluids
compatibility	osmolarity
extravasation	plasma
hemolytic reaction	plasma expanders
high-alert medication	precipitate
hypertonic solutions	replacement fluids
hypotonic solutions	Rh system

4-1 Introduction

Often, patients need only small amounts of IV fluids to keep a vein open for intermittent medication administration, for blood administration, or for diagnostic procedures. However, a patient who suffers a fluid loss that cannot adequately be replaced by oral fluids will need IV fluid to restore and then maintain the body's fluid balance. An IV fluid solution is selected for its concentration, or **osmolarity,** which affects the body's intracellular fluid (ICF) and extracellular fluid (ECF). ICF and ECF, also referred to as

TABLE 4-1 Commonly Used Abbreviations for IV Solutions

D5W	5% dextrose in water
D10W	10% dextrose in water
NS, NSS	Normal saline (0.9% NaCl)
D5 NS	5% dextrose in normal saline
Ringer's	Ringer's solution
LR or RL	Lactated Ringer's or Ringer's lactate
D5 LR	5% dextrose in lactated Ringer's
½ NS, ½ NSS	Half normal saline solution (0.45% NaCl)
⅓ NS, ⅓ NSS	One-third normal saline solution (0.33% NaCl)
¼ NS, ¼ NSS	One-fourth normal saline solution (0.225% NaCl)

Figure 4-1 IV fluids are labeled by the manufacturer with the name and exact amount of components in the solution.

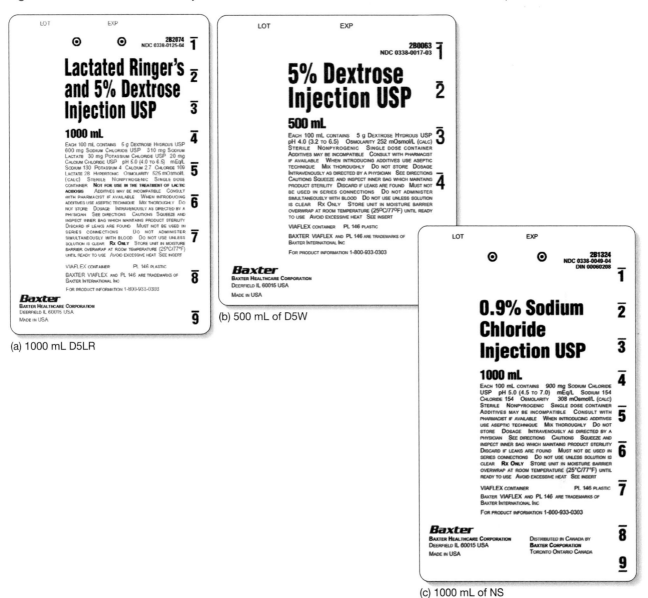

(a) 1000 mL D5LR

(b) 500 mL of D5W

(c) 1000 mL of NS

serum, normally have the same osmolarity of approximately 300 milliosmoles/liter [mOsm/l]. Patients who are overloaded with fluids have a lower serum osmolarity, and patients who are dehydrated have a higher serum osmolarity.

IV solutions are labeled with the name and exact amount of all components in the solution. Solutions contain different concentrations of dextrose (glucose) or sodium chloride (NaCl) (Figure 4-1). For example, a solution of 5% dextrose contains 5 g of dextrose per 100 mL. Normal saline (NS) is 0.9% NaCl; it contains 900 mg, or 0.9 g, of sodium chloride per 100 mL. In turn, 0.45% NaCl, or ½ NS, has 450 mg of sodium chloride per 100 mL. Other sodium chloride concentrations include 0.3% NaCl (⅓ NS), with 300 mg of sodium chloride, and 0.225% NaCl (¼ NS), with 225 mg of sodium chloride. Table 4-1 summarizes the abbreviations often used for IV solutions.

1. Describe what happens to the serum osmolarity when a patient is dehydrated.

   _____

   _____

2. Describe what happens to the serum osmolarity when a patient has a fluid overload.

   _____

   _____

3. What do the following abbreviations represent: NS, LR, D?

   _____

   _____

4-2 Types and Uses of IV Fluids

There are three categories of IV solutions: isotonic, hypertonic, and hypotonic (Figure 4-2). **Isotonic solutions** have the same concentration, or osmolarity, that serum and other body fluids do. They expand the intravascular compartment of the body without causing a shift in fluids. Isotonic solutions

Figure 4-2 Fluids move from an area of low concentration to an area of high concentration (osmosis) to achieve fluid balance.
(a) Isotonic fluids have the same concentration as blood, so the fluid does not flow into or out of the intravascular space.

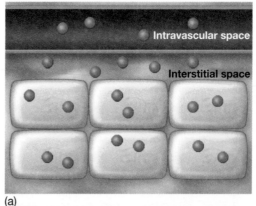
(a)

(b) Hypotonic fluids have a lower concentration than blood, so fluid moves into the cells.

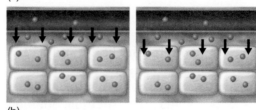
(b)

(c) Hypertonic fluids have a higher concentration than blood, so fluids leak out of the cells.

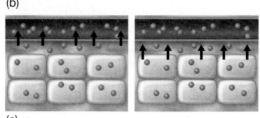
(c)

can provide hydration in patients who are dehydrated or can replace extracellular fluid losses in patients who have suffered blood loss. Isotonic solutions are also given to treat hypernatremia (sodium excess). Patients who receive isotonic solutions, especially patients with hypertension or heart failure, must be watched for fluid overload. Because isotonic solutions do not provide adequate calories and can even lead to protein loss, they should not be given for extended periods to patients who cannot eat. Common isotonic solutions are D5W, normal saline, and lactated Ringer's.

Hypertonic solutions have an osmolarity that is higher than that of serum. When infused, a hypertonic solution initially causes an increase in the osmolarity of the serum, and it pulls fluid from cells and interstitial compartments into the intravascular space. This action increases extracellular volume and causes cells to shrink. Hypertonic solutions reduce the risk of edema, stabilize blood pressure, and assist in regulating urine output. They are given to treat gastric fluid loss from diarrhea, vomiting, or nasogastric suctioning, and they are given as a temporary treatment for circulatory insufficiency and shock. Hypertonic solutions can be used to reverse the dehydration caused by overinfusion of hypotonic solutions. However, because hypertonic solutions greatly expand the intravascular space, patients receiving this solution must be monitored for circulatory overload. Hypertonic solutions are not appropriate for patients with impaired heart or kidney function. Examples of hypertonic solutions are D10W, D5 ½ NS, and D5 NS.

The third category is **hypotonic solutions.** These solutions have an osmolarity that is lower than that of serum. When administered, they cause a shift of fluids out of the intravascular space into the cells and interstitial spaces where the osmolarity is higher. Cells become hydrated, and circulating volume is decreased. Hypotonic fluids are used when the patient is dehydrated due to diuretics. Because hypotonic fluids increase extracellular fluids, they should not be given to patients with cerebral edema or increased intracranial pressure, burns, trauma, or low serum protein levels from malnutrition or liver disease. The most common hypotonic IV fluid is ½ NS.

In general, patients with normal electrolyte levels are likely to receive isotonic solutions, patients with high electrolyte levels will receive hypotonic solutions, and patients with low electrolyte levels will receive hypertonic solutions. Here are some examples:

- Patient A is a 35-year-old, healthy female who will have an IV infusion during a diagnostic test. She will require an isotonic solution such as NS.

- Patient B is an 8-year-old female who has been vomiting and has had diarrhea for 24 hours and is dehydrated. She will require a hypotonic solution such as ½ NS (0.45% NaCl) to restore the proper fluid level in her cells and tissues.

- Patient C is a 50-year-old male with burns over 35 percent of his body. He will require a hypertonic solution such as 5% dextrose and .9% NaCl (D5 NS) to pull fluid from his cells into his circulating volume as a treatment for hypovolemic shock.

Table 4-2 contains a brief summary of each of the most common IV solutions. The sections that follow describe these solutions in more detail.

TABLE 4-2 Common IV Solutions

Solution	Category	Uses/Advantages	Disadvantages
Sodium Chloride Solutions			
0.225% NaCl (¼ NS)	Hypotonic	• ECF replacement when chloride loss is greater than or equal to sodium loss • Treatment for sodium depletion • Only solution that can be used with blood products	• Possible hypernatremia • Possible depletion of other electrolytes (such as potassium) • Possible circulatory overload due to expansion of the ECF compartment
0.45% NaCl(½ NS)	Hypotonic		
0.9% NaCl(NS)	Isotonic		
3% and 5% NaCl	Hypertonic		
Dextrose Solutions			
5% dextrose in water (D5W)	Isotonic	• Calories in the form of carbohydrates • Free water • Treatment for hyperkalemia and dehydration • Vehicle for medication administration	• Blood vessel irritation, especially in higher concentrations • Dehydration caused by rapid infusion of hypertonic solutions • Possible hyperinsulinemia • Incompatibility with blood products and some medications
10% dextrose in water (D10W)	Hypertonic		
20% to 70% dextrose in water	Hypertonic		
Solutions with a Combination of Sodium Chloride and Dextrose			
5% dextrose and .225% NaCl (D5 ¼ NS)	Isotonic	• Temporary treatment of hypovolemic shock • Replacement of nutrients and electrolytes • Hydration of patients to assess kidney function • Treatment of dehydration; promotion of diuresis	• Possible hypernatremia, acidosis, and circulatory overload • Necessity of careful administration in patients with cardiac, renal, or liver disease
5% dextrose and .45% NaCl (D5 ½ NS)	Hypertonic		
5% dextrose and .9% NaCl (D5 NS)	Hypertonic		
Electrolyte Solutions			
Ringer's solution	Isotonic	• Treatment of dehydration; restoration of fluid balance presurgery and postsurgery • Toleration by patients with liver disease • Short-term blood replacement • Similarity to normal saline, with the addition of potassium and calcium	• Lack of calories • Exacerbation of sodium retention, congestive heart failure, and renal insufficiency • Contraindication in renal failure
Lactated Ringer's or Ringer's lactate (LR or RL)	Isotonic	• Treatment of all forms of dehydration, fluid losses from burns, mild metabolic acidosis, and salicylate (aspirin) overdose • Similarity to body's extracellular electrolyte content • Precursor of bicarbonate	• Possible hypernatremia • Contraindicated in patients with liver disease, hypovolemia, profound shock, or cardiac failure

Sodium Chloride Solutions

Sodium chloride (NaCl) solutions are available in a variety of concentrations. Normal saline (NS), which is 0.9% NaCl, has sodium and chloride levels that are slightly higher than the normal plasma levels of these electrolytes, but normal saline is still considered an isotonic solution. Hypotonic sodium chloride solutions, 0.45% NaCl, safely supply normal daily amounts of salt and water, whereas hypertonic sodium chloride solutions, 3% or 5% NaCl, correct severe sodium loss and water overload. Sodium chloride solutions are used to treat a variety of clinical conditions, including shock and hyponatremia (low serum sodium). In addition, sodium chloride solutions are used for fluid challenges, for replacement in diabetic ketoacidosis, and for resuscitation in trauma emergencies and are infused with blood transfusions. Because sodium chloride solutions replace ECF and can lead to fluid overload, patients with congestive heart failure (CHF), edema, or hyponatremia must be carefully monitored for such complications during infusions, especially hypertonic infusions.

Dextrose Solutions

An adult on bed rest needs approximately 1600 calories per day. If the patient has a fever or other symptoms that can cause an increase in metabolism, even more calories are required. When carbohydrate needs are not met, the body will use fat or protein stores to produce needed calories. Dextrose solutions provide calories as carbohydrates. However, lower concentrations of dextrose do not provide adequate calories: D5W supplies only 17 calories per 100 mL (170 cal/L) and D10W supplies 34 calories per 100 mL (340 cal/L). Patients could not tolerate the amount of fluids required for adequate calories in a 24-hour period. Higher concentrations of dextrose (hypertonic solutions) are available to better supply carbohydrates (see Table 4-2), but these solutions must be infused slowly through larger veins via a central line to avoid irritation of the blood vessels.

Dextrose solutions, which provide free water in addition to calories, can be used for the administration of medications and for the treatment of hyperkalemia (high serum potassium) and dehydration. When infused too rapidly, solutions with higher concentrations of dextrose can cause cellular dehydration by pulling fluid from the interstitial space into the ECF. Infusions of the higher dextrose concentrations should not be stopped suddenly; they must be decreased slowly over 48 hours. Otherwise, the additional carbohydrates provided by the solution will cause the patient's pancreas to excrete too much insulin.

Solutions with a Combination of Sodium Chloride and Dextrose

Solutions with a combination of sodium chloride and dextrose prevent some of the adverse effects that occur when sodium chloride or dextrose is administered separately. Because combination solutions provide more water than is required for excretion of sodium, they make good hydrating solutions. Combination solutions are a good choice for fluid replacement in patients with excessive loss of fluid due to sweating, vomiting, or gastric suction. Patients with heart, kidney, or liver diseases must be monitored closely to prevent fluid overload.

Multiple Electrolyte Solutions

Multiple electrolyte solutions are used as replacement fluids or maintenance fluids, depending on the solution's concentration of electrolytes. **Replacement fluids** replace electrolytes or fluids lost because of dehydration, hemorrhage, vomiting, or diarrhea. Some solutions are specifically formulated to replace electrolytes lost by vomiting or gastric suctioning. These solutions may contain lactate or acetate to treat metabolic acidosis, which is a disruption of the body's acid-base balance. This disruption may be due to an accumulation of acid without enough bicarbonate or to a loss of bicarbonate. Either condition results in the inability of the body to neutralize the effects of the acid. Metabolic acidosis may develop from alcoholism, starvation (ketoacidosis), or a lack of insulin. It may also be caused by respiratory or circulatory failure, renal failure, or the ingestion of certain drugs or toxins such as salicylates or ethylene glycol. **Maintenance fluids** maintain the balance of fluids and electrolytes in patients. Multiple electrolyte solutions are recommended for use in patients with trauma, fluid losses in the gastrointestinal tract, dehydration, sodium loss, acidosis, and burns. To avoid complications, the health care professional must carefully assess patient status prior to starting a multiple electrolyte solution.

Plasma Expanders

Plasma expanders act osmotically to expand the intravascular space. They are used to rapidly increase circulating volume in emergencies. Two forms of plasma expanders are blood products and albumin; there are also synthetic forms such as dextran, mannitol, and hetastarch. *Dextran* can be used to treat shock due to trauma, burns, or hemorrhage, but it is not a substitute for blood or blood products. Complications from dextran include **anaphylaxis** (a life-threatening allergic reaction with hypotension and severe respiratory distress), fluid overload, and dilution of electrolytes. *Mannitol* is a sugar alcohol substance that removes excess body fluids. It promotes diuresis and excretion of toxic substances and is used to treat increased intracranial pressure and cerebral edema. Complications include fluid and electrolyte imbalances, cellular dehydration, fluid overload, and nervous system toxicity. *Hetastarch* is similar to albumin. When hetastarch is given, fluid is pulled from the cells into the intravascular space. Hetastarch is used to replace fluids in the treatment of shock caused by decreased circulating volume. Complications include anaphylaxis, altered platelet function, volume overload, fluid and electrolyte imbalances, and decreased hematocrit and plasma proteins caused by increased fluid volume. *Albumin* is a natural plasma protein obtained from blood. Its action is similar to that of the other plasma expanders, and albumin may also increase plasma protein volume. It is used to treat shock related to circulating volume deficit, to provide protein, and to bind bilirubin. Complications include fluid overload, anemia, bleeding, dilution or depletion of electrolytes, and allergic reactions.

Five percent (5%) sodium bicarbonate solution is used to neutralize excess acids and to restore balance in patients with metabolic acidosis or severe hyperkalemia (high potassium). Metabolic alkalosis, hypocalcemia (low calcium), hypokalemia (low potassium), hypovolemia (low blood volume), and sodium retention are complications of bicarbonate infusions. Infiltration can result in damage to tissues, causing cellulitis, necrosis, and ulceration. Alcohol solutions are hypertonic mixtures of 5% ethyl alcohol and 5% dextrose in water. They are metabolized by the liver and are used to replace water and to provide calories. Complications are related to continuous use or rapid infusion and include hypervolemia, intoxication, dilution of electrolytes, and acid-base imbalances. Infiltration causes phlebitis and tissue necrosis. Alcohol solutions should not be administered to patients with a history of alcoholism.

Blood and Blood Products

Blood is the body's main transport system for oxygen, nutrients, hormones, and other important substances. The adult body contains about 5 liters of blood. When a patient experiences a decrease in circulating blood volume, replacement of blood or blood products may be necessary. Any decrease in circulating volume disrupts the body's fluid and electrolyte balance. Infusing blood or blood products restores circulating volume, improves the ability of the blood to carry oxygen, and replaces **blood components** that the body is deficient in, including factors that enable blood to clot. Blood components that can be infused are whole blood, packed red blood cells (RBCs), leukocyte-poor RBCs, platelets, and fresh frozen plasma (see Table 4-3).

Blood is composed of plasma and cells. **Plasma,** the liquid component of blood, is about 55 percent of blood volume and consists of water (serum), protein, lipids (fats), electrolytes, vitamins, carbohydrates, bilirubin, nonprotein nitrogen compounds, and gases. The cellular portion of blood is composed of erythrocytes (red blood cells, or RBCs), leukocytes (white blood cells, or WBCs) and thrombocytes (platelets). Blood deficiencies can be corrected by infusion of whole blood or individual components.

Transfused blood may be autologous (from the recipient) or from a donor. Autologous blood decreases the risks associated with transfusions but may not be available, especially in emergencies. Donor blood is more readily available but must be carefully screened and tested to ensure safety (Figure 4-3). In addition, donor blood must be typed and cross-matched for compatibility with the recipient to prevent a **hemolytic reaction** that may occur when the donor blood and recipient are mismatched. Red blood cells carry an inherited antigen that can initiate an immune response and the formation of a corresponding antibody if the recipient does not carry the antigen. The interaction of the antigen and antibody can cause agglutination, or clumping of blood cells.

ABO Blood Groups

Blood groups are identified by their antigens: A, B, AB, and O (carries neither A nor B antigens). The antigens are found on the red blood cells. This grouping is known as the **ABO system**. Type A blood carries anti-B antibodies, B carries anti-A antibodies, AB carries neither antibody, and O carries both anti-A and anti-B antibodies the antibodies will react with the antigens. Because type AB blood carries neither antibody, a person with this blood type can receive blood from any of the four groups. Such a person is called a *universal recipient*. Type O blood does not have either A or B antigens and can be transfused in an emergency to any patient regardless of the recipient's blood type. A person with Type O blood, then, is a *universal donor*. Table 4-4 offers a summary of compatible blood types.

TABLE 4-3 Blood and Blood Products

Blood Component	Volume	Compatibility Requirement	Key Points
Whole blood	450–500 mL	• Must be ABO- and Rh-compatible.	• Is used to restore blood volume for victims with trauma, burns, or blood loss greater than 25% of total blood volume. • Is contraindicated if loss can be managed by blood components and plasma expanders. • May result in fluid overload and hyperkalemia due to cell breakdown during storage.
Packed RBCs	250–350 mL	• Should be ABO-compatible. • Group O may be given in an emergency until ABO typing is complete. • Must be Rh-compatible.	• Is used to improve the oxygen-carrying capacity in anemic patients by increasing the number of circulating RBCs. • Increases RBC mass without increasing fluid volume.
Leukocyte- poor RBCs	200 mL	• Should be ABO-compatible. • Group O may be given in an emergency until ABO typing is complete. • Must be Rh-compatible.	• Is the same component as packed RBCs except that most of the leukocytes have been removed. • Has the same uses as the packed RBCs component does. • Is less likely to cause febrile reactions, because leukocytes have been removed. • Can be used to treat immunosuppressed patients.
Platelets	40–70 mL	• ABO match is not required but is recommended for repeated transfusions. • Rh compatibility is recommended.	• Is used to treat thrombocytopenia (low platelet count) due to decreased production of platelets, destruction or massive transfusion of whole stored blood, or abnormal platelet function. • May be pooled in one bag even if from random donors.
Fresh frozen plasma	200–250 mL	• Must be ABO-compatible.	• Is given to increase and/or replace clotting factors and to counteract the effects of warfarin therapy. • Must be used within 24 hours of thawing.

Hemolytic reactions can be life threatening and may occur with as little as 10 mL of blood or blood product. The reaction occurs because antibodies to the antigens attach to the surface of red cells and cause them to clump together. Activated by the antigen-antibody reaction, the body's immune system causes destruction of the red blood cells, releasing hemoglobin into the blood, which can damage renal tubules and lead to renal failure. Symptoms of a transfusion reaction include headache, chest pain, chills, back pain, and fever.

Figure 4-3 Transfused blood or blood products may be autologous (from the recipient) or from a donor. Pictured here is O⁺ blood. O blood is the universal donor.

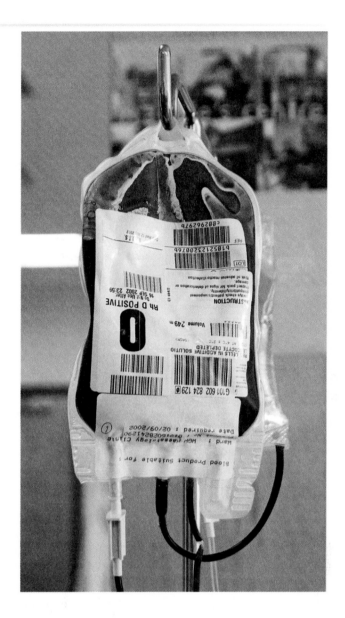

Rh Factor

The Rh (Rhesus) factor is another major inherited blood antigen. Blood is either Rh-positive or Rh-negative. Rh postive has Rh antigens. Rh negative does not. The blood donor and recipient should be matched for the Rh factor. This matching is known as the **Rh system.** Initial exposure of an Rh-negative

TABLE 4-4 Recipient Blood Group and Compatible Types

Recipient Blood Group	Compatible Donor Group
A	A, O
B	B, O
AB	AB, A, B, O
O	O

recipient to Rh-positive blood generally does not cause a reaction. However, anti-Rh antibodies that form as a result of this initial exposure may cause hemolytic reactions if more Rh-positive blood is transfused.

Blood Transfusions

In addition to the major antigens and antibodies of the ABO system and the Rh system, other antigens and antibodies may be introduced during blood transfusions and may cause transfusion reactions. Every patient's blood sample and blood product must be carefully cross-matched to prevent transfusion reactions. In most states, an RN must hang blood and blood products; however, as a health care professional, you may be asked to participate in verification and patient identification prior to initiation of the transfusion.

Safety and Infection Control

Transfuse with Normal Saline Only

Blood and blood products are transfused only with normal saline. No other medications or solutions may be given through the same IV tubing.

Checkpoint Questions 4-2

1. List the three categories of IV fluids based on osmolarity. How are the three types different?

   _____

   _____

2. What is the importance of the ABO and Rh systems?

   _____

   _____

 Before you continue to the next section, answer the previous Checkpoint Questions and complete the Types and Uses of IV Fluids activity under Chapter 4 on the student CD.

4-3 Additives

Patients may need additional infusions that are not a normal part of commercially available products. Patients with a critically high glucose level, for example, may require additional electrolytes such as potassium or insulin. Intravenous administration can provide some or all nutritional requirements for patients unable to obtain adequate nutrition orally or enterally (directly into the gastrointestinal tract).

Parenteral Nutrition

Parenteral nutrition is the IV infusion of nutrients, including amino acids, dextrose, fat, electrolytes, vitamins, and trace elements (see Table 4-5). Parenteral nutrition solutions may be administered peripherally or through a central vein. Peripherally administered solutions are less concentrated

TABLE 4-5 Components of Parenteral Nutrition Solutions

Component	Purpose
Dextrose or dextrose substitutes	• Dextrose provides calories needed for energy. • Solutions can be 5% to 70% dextrose.
Amino acids	• Protein is added to replace essential amino acids, maintain protein stores, and prevent protein loss from muscles.
Electrolytes	• The patient's lab test results and metabolic needs are used to determine which electrolytes are added. • Electrolytes necessary for long-term total parenteral nutrition are potassium, magnesium, calcium, sodium chloride, and phosphorous.
Vitamins	• Fat- and water-soluble vitamins, biotin, and folic acid are added to meet daily requirements.
Micronutrients	• Trace elements promote normal metabolism and include zinc, copper, chromium, selenium, and manganese.
Water	• The amount of water added is based on individual needs.
Insulin	• Insulin is often added to counteract hyperglycemia caused by the high concentration of glucose in the solution.
Fats	• Lipid emulsions are a concentrated source of energy and prevent or correct fatty acid deficiencies. • Lipid emulsions are administered in a separate infusion.

and provide only partial nutritional requirements. Infusions through central veins can be more highly concentrated and, therefore, can provide the patient's total nutritional requirements.

Peripheral parenteral nutrition (PPN) may be used to help a patient meet minimum calorie and protein needs if the patient does not need to gain weight. PPN requires lower concentrations of dextrose and amino acids to decrease the risk of damage to peripheral veins. The dextrose concentration should not be greater than 10% to prevent sclerosing (hardening) of veins. Because of the risk of phlebitis and infiltrations, PPN therapy is difficult to maintain and is therefore not appropriate for long-term therapy. Contraindications include severe malnourishment, lack of tolerance for large fluid volumes, poor or inaccessible peripheral veins, nutritional needs greater than what can be met by PPN, and a functional gastrointestinal tract.

Total parenteral nutrition (TPN) is needed to restore or maintain nutritional status in patients with illnesses or injuries that have led to a decrease in or absence of oral intake, resulting in weight loss and decreased caloric and protein levels. Multiple trauma injuries, severe burns, and gastrointestinal disorders that reduce or prevent absorption are some reasons that a patient may require TPN. TPN may be used for long-term nutritional support, but it must be administered through a central venous access because of the concentration of the solution, about six times that of blood. Infusion rates are initially low and are increased gradually to allow the body to adjust to the higher glucose levels. The patient's blood glucose should be monitored, and insulin can be added to the TPN solution if necessary. Because of the high dextrose content, TPN should never be stopped abruptly. Instead, the infusion rate should be gradually decreased over 24 hours to prevent rebound hypoglycemia. Contraindications include a functional gastrointestinal tract, inability to obtain IV access, poor patient prognosis not justifying aggressive nutritional support, TPN nutrition that would last less than five days, and risks that outweigh the benefits.

Heparin

Heparin infusions are used to prevent and treat various thromboembolic (blood-clotting) disorders such as deep vein thrombosis, pulmonary embolism, and atrial fibrillation with clotting. Heparin does not dissolve clots but instead keeps clots from expanding and prevents development of new ones. Heparin should be administered via an infusion pump. Dosage calculations and pump settings must be verified by a second person. Infusion rates are closely monitored, and titration is based on the patient's PT/INR. The prothrombin time, or protime (PT), measures how long it takes for the patient's blood to clot, but because results may vary from lab to lab, a ratio called the international normalized ratio (INR) is used to standardize the results. This test may be done by a laboratory, on a clinical unit, or in the doctor's office. If the PT/INR is prolonged, the patient is at greater risk for bleeding.

Heparin is a high-alert medication and carries an increased risk for causing significant patient harm when used incorrectly (Figure 4-4). All health care personnel should be informed when a patient they are caring for is receiving heparin infusions. Watch your patients on heparin closely for signs of bleeding and hemorrhage. Apply pressure to venipunctures and injection sites to prevent bleeding or hematoma formation at the site. Be especially careful when giving mouth care, shaving male patients, and performing other tasks that could cause bleeding.

Patient Education & Communication **Anticoagulant Therapy**

Instruct patients who are receiving heparin or other anticoagulant therapy to report any unusual bruising or bleeding. Tell them to watch for and report bloody or black tarry stools, nosebleeds, or blood in the urine.

Troubleshooting **Patients Receiving Heparin**

You are assigned to a patient receiving a heparin infusion through an infusion pump. At the shift report, the health care professional said that the patient's PT/INR was prolonged so the heparin was held for 2 hours and the rate was decreased when it was restarted. You know that you need to watch for signs of bleeding and hemorrhage.

What should you look for? How will this patient's condition affect the care that you provide?

_____

_____

Insulin

Diabetic patients who are in ketoacidosis, an emergency condition of acidosis due to high glucose levels, are treated with infusions of low-dose regular insulin. Patients receiving insulin infusions must be closely monitored for hypoglycemia. Their blood glucose is checked frequently with a blood glucose meter to guide changes in the infusion rate. Initially, the insulin is infused in a solution of either 0.9% NaCl or 0.45% NaCl. Once the patient's blood glucose lowers to near 250 mg/dl, dextrose is added to the infusion to maintain this blood sugar level for 12 to 24 hours. Adding dextrose prevents complications from a too-rapid lowering of the blood sugar. The patient is converted to subcutaneous insulin once the acidosis is corrected, vital signs are normalized, and oral intake is tolerated. Insulin is also a high-alert medication and carries an increased risk for causing significant patient harm when used incorrectly.

Figure 4-4 Heparin and insulin are both considered high-alert medications because they will most likely cause injury if misused.

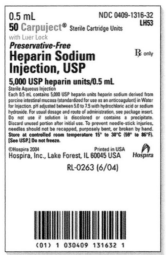

(a)

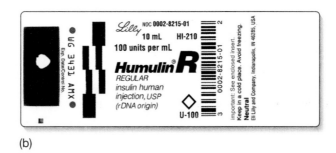

(b)

 Troubleshooting **Patients Receiving Insulin**

A patient assigned to you today was admitted last evening because of very high glucose levels and had been put on an insulin drip. No changes have been made to the rate of the drip since the patient was admitted. When you check the patient after hearing and reviewing herreport, you find that she is confused and her skin is cool and moist.

What should you do? What do you think is happening to this patient?

_____

_____

Electrolytes and Vitamins

Electrolytes are added to IV solutions to replace patient losses. Potassium, magnesium, phosphorus, and calcium are usually added to a large-volume IV bag; however, they may be given in smaller volumes via a secondary set as an IV piggyback (IVPB). The selection and amount of electrolytes are based on the patient's renal and cardiac function, acid-base balance, electrolyte deficiencies, and disease-specific needs. IV bags, especially ones containing potassium, should be gently shaken back and forth prior to infusion to prevent the patient from getting a large dose right at the beginning of the infusion. Potassium is irritating to the vein, so IV sites must be closely monitored for phlebitis and infiltration. To avoid **precipitate** formation, IV calcium is not given with bicarbonate solutions (a precipitate is when a solid substance forms in a solution and creates a sediment); also, IV calcium can cause severe tissue damage if infiltration occurs. Magnesium and phosphorus are normally added to TPN solutions, not administered as separate infusions.

Some diseases change the vitamin requirements that the body needs for growth, maintenance, and metabolic processes. Vitamins can be added to supplemental preparations or can be administered separately for specific deficiencies. Vitamin K is not part of many commercial preparations, so it may need to be added separately. Vitamin C promotes wound healing, so an extra amount may be added to the IV of a patient with a wound that is healing poorly. Folic acid may be administered for macrocytic anemia (*macrocytic* means abnormally large RBCs). Patients with a history of alcohol abuse may require additional amounts of folic acid and thiamine (Vitamin B_{12}) to correct deficiencies associated with this disease. B vitamins support the metabolism of carbohydrates and the maintenance of gastrointestinal function, two processes that are important for postoperative patients.

Safety and Infection Control

Safety for the Elderly

Because of the normal aging process, elderly patients are more likely to develop fluid and electrolyte disorders. Fluid replacement in the elderly requires close monitoring to prevent fluid overloads that can lead to electrolyte imbalances. IV therapy for elderly patients should always be administered with an IV infusion pump.

Checkpoint Questions 4-3

1. What is parenteral nutrition?

   _____

   _____

2. If heparin does not dissolve clots that have already formed, what is its therapeutic effect?

   _____

   _____

3. What potential problems could occur when the electrolyte potassium is added to an IV solution? What problems could occur when calcium is added?

   _____

   _____

Before you continue to the next section, answer the previous Checkpoint Questions and complete the IV Additives activity under Chapter 4 on the student CD.

4-4 Compatibility

To ensure a therapeutic response to the therapy, the components of an IV solution must be compatible. **Compatibility** means the ability to be mixed and administered without undesirable chemical or physical changes or the loss of therapeutic effect. The additive—whether a vitamin, electrolyte, or medication—must be compatible with the diluent (liquid used to reconstitute the medication) and with the solution used to deliver the medication. Factors affecting drug compatibility include

- The order in which drugs are mixed
- Drug concentrations
- The length of time that drugs are in contact with other drugs or solutions
- Temperature
- Exposure to light
- pH

An **incompatibility** occurs when the additives of a solution react or interact to change the expected action. Incompatibilities may cause loss of therapeutic effects of the solution or medication. The three types of incompatibilities are physical, chemical, and therapeutic.

Chemical incompatibility is the result of changes in either the medication or the solution. Drug concentration, pH of the solution, time, temperature, and light are all factors associated with chemical incompatibilities. To avoid changes that may occur with time, no IV solution should hang longer than 24 hours. Chemical incompatibilities may or may not be visible and may simply result in the deterioration of the drug. An example of a visible change is the color change that occurs in nitroprusside (a light-sensitive antihypertensive medication) when it is exposed to light. Nitroprusside solutions are normally slightly brown, but prolonged exposure to light can cause the color to change to dark brown, orange, blue, green, or dark red and can necessitate disposal of the bag. To prevent color change in nitroprusside, the IV bag should be protected with aluminum foil or similar product.

A physical incompatibility occurs when multiple drugs are added to a solution or when a drug is added to an inappropriate solution. The incompatible mixture produces a solution that is not safe to infuse. A physical incompatibility may cause the formation of precipitate (sediment) that is visible or is too small to detect. The solution may become hazy or cloudy or develop gas bubbles. Calcium or sodium bicarbonate in a solution, for example, increases the chance that a precipitate will form.

Therapeutic incompatibility is an undesirable reaction that may occur when two or more drugs are given together. One medication may increase or inhibit the effects of another medication. The only indication of a therapeutic incompatibility may be when the patient fails to exhibit the expected clinical response to the medications. Some antibiotics, for example, are therapeutically incompatible and should not be infused at the same time or through the same tubing.

Some common incompatible medications and solutions are

- Ampicillin in D5W
- Cefotaxime sodium mixed with sodium bicarbonate
- Diazepam mixed with potassium chloride
- Dopamine hydrochloride mixed with sodium bicarbonate
- Penicillin mixed with heparin
- Penicillin mixed with vitamin B complex
- Sodium bicarbonate in lactated Ringer's
- Tetracycline hydrochloride mixed with calcium chloride

Before you mix or infuse medications and/or IV fluids, check their compatibility using a compatibility chart, a drug reference book, the Internet, the pharmacy, or the package insert. Carefully inspect the IV solution and the tubing for cloudiness or crystals. The following actions will help you avoid incompatibility problems:

- Change solutions every 24 hours
- Carefully check IV bags before hanging them
- Do not infuse a solution that is cloudy or forms a precipitate
- Select the correct diluent to reconstitute the drug
- Do not mix drugs that have a special diluent with other drugs
- Select the correct solution for the infusion
- Flush the IV line between infusions of incompatible medications
- Follow the manufacturer's recommendations

Checkpoint Question 4-4

1. What factors affect compatibility?

_____

_____

 Before you continue to the next section, answer the previous Checkpoint Question and complete the Compatibility activity under Chapter 4 on the student CD.

4-5 Common IV Medications

Approximately 40 percent of the medications administered in the hospital setting are given intravenously. IV medications are ordered when a patient is unable to take oral medications, when a patient cannot absorb medications through the gastrointestinal tract, or when a patient's condition requires a rapid therapeutic response. The IV administration of medication has numerous advantages. IV-administered medications produce rapid results, which is often necessary during emergencies. Medications introduced directly into the bloodstream reach therapeutic levels quickly and often at lower doses than would be needed for other routes. Dosages are easily adjusted by changing the concentration of the medication in the solution or by changing the administration rate. If an adverse reaction occurs, administration can be

TABLE 4-6 IV Medication Administration

Advantages	Disadvantages
• Direct access to the circulatory system	• Drug/solution incompatibilities
• Available route for patients unable to tolerate oral medications	• Absorption by IV bag or administration set, which decreases the amount of medication administered
• Fewer needlesticks, so is less painful for patients than are IM or SQ routes	• Errors in mixing techniques
• A means for rapid drug action and therapeutic response	• Speed shock if medication or solution is infused too rapidly
• Control over rate of administration	• Phlebitis
• A means for immediate discontinuation of drug administration if an adverse reaction occurs	• Extravasation caused by vesicant drugs

stopped immediately, thereby limiting the amount of medication absorbed by the patient. This rapid response to a problem is not possible with other routes of administration. The IV administration of medication is generally less painful for the patient than are subcutaneous (sub-Q) or intramuscular (IM) routes because the IV route does not require frequent injections.

Administering medications by the IV route also has several disadvantages. Incompatibility issues, discussed in the previous section, may occur. An error can be made when the medication is reconstituted or added to the IV solution. The patient may develop phlebitis or extravasation when irritant drugs are administered or if the IV is not seated securely in the vein. Phlebitis is inflammation of the vein, and **extravasation** is when IV solutions or medications leak into the tissue surrounding the IV site. If the medication or solution is infused too rapidly, the patient may experience signs of shock: dizziness, flushing, headache, tightness in the chest, hypotension, and irregular pulse. This speed shock can be avoided by using microdrip sets, using an infusion pump, and carefully monitoring the infusion rate. Table 4-6 provides a summary of the advantages and disadvantages of IV administration of medication.

In the inpatient setting, IV medications are often prepared by the pharmacy and delivered to the patient unit. Prior to administering premixed medications, carefully compare the label on the container to the physician's order. Inspect the solution for precipitates or changes in color or clarity. Medications that are not prepared by the pharmacy are mixed by a health care professional just prior to administration. Powdered medications will need to be reconstituted. The package insert provides information about reconstituting.

Classification of Medications

Medications can be classified in several ways. They are sometimes classified by generic/trade name. The generic name of a medication is based on its chemical composition and is the name most often used in the inpatient setting. The trade name of a medication is the name that is copyrighted by the pharmaceutical company that markets the medication. A generic drug

TABLE 4-7 Classification of Medications

Classification	Purpose
Anti-infectives • Antibiotics • Antifungals • Antivirals	Prevent or treat bacterial, fungal, or viral infections by destroying or inhibiting the growth of infecting organism
Cardiovascular Medications • Antiarrhythmic drugs	• Used to restore the normal heart rate and rhythm and to preserve regular ventricular rhythm
• Congestive heart failure agents • Contractility agents • Diuretics • Vasodilators	 • Improve cardiac contractions • Decrease circulating volume • Decrease the pressure that the heart has to pump against to expel blood
• Antihypertensives	• Used to safely lower the blood pressure
• Anticoagulants • Thrombolytics	• Limit or prevent blood clots • Dissolve blood clots
Central Nervous System Medications • Anticonvulsants • Narcotic analgesics • Sedatives • Anxiolytic agents	 • Control seizures • Prevent or relieve pain • Provide a calming effect • Lessen anxiety
Gastrointestinal Medications • Antiulcer medications • H_2 blockers • Proton pump inhibitors • Antiemetics	 • Reduce acid secretion in the stomach • Control nausea and vomiting
Chemotherapeutic Agents	Treat cancer; are categorized according to their action on cell production
• Antimetabolites and vinca alkaloids	• Inhibit mitosis (cell division) or interfere with DNA synthesis, thereby preventing reproduction
• Alkylating agents, antitumor antibiotics, and nitrosoureas	• Interfere with or inhibit DNA replication, synthesis, or repair

may be produced by more than one company and, therefore, may have more than one trade name. For example, acetaminophen is a generic name, and Tylenol, Tempra, and Liquiprin are all trade names for acetaminophen. Medications can also be classified simply as prescription or nonprescription (over-the-counter drugs). However, the most common classification of medications and the one used in this textbook is the functional or therapeutic classification (see Table 4-7). This classification refers to the clinical indication for administering the medication (e.g., antihypertensives, laxatives),

Figure 4-5 One type of anti-infective IV medication is Fortaz.

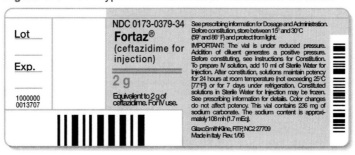

the body system affected by the medication (e.g., the gastrointestinal tract), or the pharmacology of the medication (e.g., barbiturates). The following sections provide information about the most commonly administered IV medications grouped by classification: anti-infectives, cardiovascular medications, central nervous system medications, gastrointestinal medications, and chemotherapy agents. A list of common IV medications can be found in Appendix C.

Anti-infectives

Anti-infectives prevent or treat bacterial, fungal, or viral infections by destroying or inhibiting the growth of the infecting organism. Anti-infectives are administered to achieve therapeutic blood levels in a patient. Several steps must be taken before a patient is administered an anti-infective. First, the source of the infection, for example an IV catheter tip, is located and the organism is identified through a culture of blood, urine, sputum, or wound material. Second, to prevent toxicity, the patient's renal and hepatic function is assessed. Third, the patient is asked about medication allergies, or the patient's record is checked for this information.

Anti-infectives include antibiotics, antifungal medications, and antiviral medications (Figure 4-5). *Antibiotics* are used to treat most common bacterial infections and are either bacteriostatic (inhibiting growth or reproduction of bacteria) or bactericidal (killing bacteria outright). The emergence of new or resistant pathogens has led to a wide selection of antibiotics. Antibiotics are grouped into eight major types: penicillins, cephalosporins, aminoglycosides, tetracyclines, erythromycins, sulfonamides, quinolones, and chloramphenicol. Some antibiotics, such as tetracyclines and erythromycins, are broad-spectrum and are effective against many different pathogens. Other antibiotics are effective against either gram-positive or gram-negative bacteria; for example, aminoglycosides are more specific to gram-negative bacteria such as *Escherichia coli* and *Pseudomonas*. Selection of the antibiotic is based on the pathogen causing the infection.

Systemic fungal infections are not as common as bacterial infections but can be difficult to treat when they do occur. They occur most frequently in immunosuppressed patients, for example, patients with AIDS or who have had organ transplants. *Antifungals* are either fungicidal (killing the fungi causing the infection) or fungistatic (stopping the growth of the fungi).

Antifungal agents are administered slowly over 2 to 6 hours. Examples of antifungals are amphotericin B and fluconazole.

Most viral infections, such as the common cold, are self-limiting (end on their own) and do not require treatment, but more serious ones, such as AIDS, do need to be treated. Immunosuppressed patients require treatment for viral infections to prevent fatal complications. *Antivirals* are selectively toxic to viruses, preventing their replication. Selection of the antiviral is based on the infecting pathogen. Acyclovir, for example, inhibits many viruses but is primarily used for serious herpes infections. Ganciclovir, although similar to acyclovir, is primarily administered to AIDS patients.

Cardiovascular Medications

Cardiovascular medications treat cardiac dysrhythmias, congestive heart failure, thromboembolic disease, and hypertension emergencies. *Antiarrhythmic drugs* are used to restore the normal heart rate and rhythm and to preserve regular ventricular rhythm. They work by changing the movement of one or more electrolytes (sodium, potassium, calcium) across the heart cells' membranes, but they also affect the ability of the heart to contract. Patients receiving IV-administered antiarrhythmic drugs must be on cardiac monitoring because of the possibility that the dysrhythmia will become worse or a new one will develop. Heart failure is the inability of the heart to pump adequate blood to satisfy the oxygen and nutrient needs of vital organs. Congestive heart failure is heart failure that has progressed over many years and in which compensatory mechanisms have started to fail. Acute exacerbations may be treated with *congestive heart failure agents* that improve contractility (digoxin), *diuretics* to decrease circulating volume (furosemide), and/or *vasodilators* (dopamine) to decrease the pressure that the heart has to pump against to expel blood.

Antihypertensives are administered to safely lower a patient's blood pressure. IV antihypertensives are usually given during hypertensive episodes—when other routes would be too slow—for effective lowering of the blood pressure to prevent complications such as stroke. A variety of antihypertensives are available that work in different ways to lower the blood pressure: beta-adrenergic blockers (metoprolol, propranolol), calcium channel blockers (verapamil, diltiazem), and angiotensin converting enzyme (ACE) inhibitors (enalapril). A vasodilator such as nitroprusside can be administered in a hypertensive emergency. Patients receiving an IV antihypertensive must be carefully monitored to prevent the blood pressure from going too low.

Anticoagulants (such as heparin, which was discussed in the section on additives) limit or prevent blood clots. *Thrombolytics* (streptokinase, alteplase) actually dissolve the clot that has formed. Thrombolytics are used in the treatment of acute heart attacks, strokes caused by a blood clot, and massive pulmonary emboli.

Central Nervous System Medications

Central nervous system medications control seizures; relieve pain; control agitation and provide sedation (lorazepam, chlordiazepoxide); and treat alcohol withdrawal (chlordiazepoxide). IV *anticonvulsants* are used when patients are unable to take oral seizure medications or when serum levels of the anticonvulsant need to be raised quickly to stop or prevent seizure activity. One example of an anticonvulsant is phenytoin, which must be mixed in 0.9% NaCl to prevent the formation of a precipitate. Phenytoin is also very irritating to tissues, so close observation of the IV site for infiltration is important. *Narcotic analgesics* are used for pain prevention or relief and are closely controlled by strict laws. IV narcotic analgesics are administered via a lockable infusion pump that can be set for patient-controlled analgesia (PCA) or continuous infusion. PCA, which was discussed in Chapter 3, allows the patient to self-administer pain medicine within prescribed limits. Patients must be closely monitored for pain level and level of consciousness. Morphine is the most common IV narcotic analgesic. *Sedatives* (phenobarbital) and *anxiolytic agents* (diazepam, lorazepam) are used to provide a calming (sedative) effect and to lessen anxiety. They are frequently given preoperatively and can be used as adjuncts to analgesic therapy. Some are used in the treatment of seizures. These drugs cause central nervous system depression, so patients must be closely monitored to prevent overmedication.

Gastrointestinal Medications

IV medications that target the gastrointestinal system include antiulcer medications and antiemetics. *Antiulcer medications* such as H_2 blockers (ranitidine) and proton pump inhibitors (omeprazole) work by reducing acid secretion in the stomach. They are used acutely to treat ulcers until the patient can tolerate oral forms. They are also used prophylactically to prevent ulcer formation in seriously ill patients. Stress ulcers can develop quickly in response to severe illnesses or injuries even if the trauma does not involve the stomach. Major burns, trauma, renal or hepatic failure, and serious respiratory disease are some stressors that can cause ulcers. Most *antiemetics* control nausea and vomiting by blocking receptors in the central nervous system that trigger these symptoms (phenergan) or by affecting gastric motility (metoclopramide). Patients on these medications must be monitored to prevent central nervous system depression, especially if they are also receiving sedatives or antihistamines.

Chemotherapeutic Agents

Chemotherapeutic agents are used in the treatment of cancer and are categorized according to their action on cell production. Cycle-specific agents, which act on the cells at various phases in the cell cycle, include *antimetabolites* (5FU, methotrexate) and *vinca alkaloids* (vincristine). These drugs inhibit mitosis (cell division) or interfere with DNA synthesis, preventing reproduction. Cycle-nonspecific agents act on cells that are not going through the division phase. These drugs interfere with or inhibit DNA replication, synthesis, or repair. Examples of cycle-nonspecific agents include *alkylating agents* (cisplatin), *antitumor antibiotics* (mitomycin), and *nitrosoureas* (carmustine).

Cancer cell type and stage determine the selection of chemotherapeutic drugs. Rapidly growing cancers such as acute leukemias respond best to cycle-specific medications because of the faster rate of cell division. Slower growing cancers such as gastrointestinal or pulmonary tumors have a slower cell division rate and, therefore, respond better to cycle-nonspecific drugs. Because tumor cells are always at various phases in the cell cycle, cancer patients often receive a combination of agents that act at different phases or target different sites on the cell. In combination, chemotherapy drugs enhance the effect of each other, so smaller doses of each can be administered, decreasing the chance of toxicity. Combination therapy also decreases the chance that the tumor cells will develop resistance to chemotherapy.

Chemotherapy treatment requires repeated doses given in repeated cycles. Cyclic treatment allows time for normal cells to regenerate, because chemotherapy drugs can also damage healthy cells. Complications of chemotherapy include but are not limited to

- Bleeding due to a decrease in platelets
- Infection due to a decrease in white blood cells
- Anemia due to a decrease in red blood cells that results in a decrease in the oxygen-carrying capacity of blood
- Anorexia and/or nausea and vomiting with risk of dehydration and poor nutritional status
- Alopecia (loss of hair)
- Stomatitis (inflammation of the oral mucosa)
- Phlebitis and sclerosing of veins

Patients receiving chemotherapeutic drugs must be closely monitored. Adjustments to treatments are based on patient response or the appearance of complications.

Administration of IV Medications

Health care professionals who are administering IV medications must follow the same care and safety practices that they would follow to administer medications given by any other route. A pharmacist should review all new medication orders, and a health care professional should verify medication orders at the time they are transcribed to the medication record and prior to administration. The health care professional verifies the following information:

- The patient's name (to ensure that the medication is transcribed on the correct record)
- The date of the order
- The name of the medication
- The dosage
- The route
- Any special instructions for administration
- The time and frequency of the medication
- The practitioner's signature

TABLE 4-8 Seven Rights of Medication Administration

Right	Explanation
Right medication	• Compare the medication label to the medication sheet three times. • Note the medication's expiration date. • Know the action, dose, and method of administration of this medication. • Know the side effects of this medication.
Right patient	• Ask the patient to state his or her name. • Verify the patient's armband for name and unique number (social security number, date of birth, or unique hospital number). The unique number must agree with the medication record.
Right time	• Know your facility's policy on medication administration time (usually 30 minutes to 1 hour before and after the time the medication was scheduled to be administered).
Right route	• Ask for a new order if you are unable to administer the medication by the route ordered.
Right method (technique)	• Use the proper technique to administer a medication by the route ordered.
Right dose	• Verify the dose with the medication record. • Double-check any calculations; have a second person verify any calculations. • Have a second person verify the administration of heparin, insulin, or digitalis. • Know the usual dose of this medication; question any dosage outside the safe range.
Right documentation	• Maintain timely and accurate records of all medications given. • Document the effects of and the patient's response to medications such as pain medications and antihypertensives. • Document any pre- or post-measurements or observations made in relation to a medication, such as blood pressure, temperature, pain score. • Document patient education as it pertains to medications.

If you are administering an IV medication, you must verify whether the patient has an allergy to the medication, especially if it is the first dose of a new medication. Because the body responds more rapidly to medications given intravenously, an allergic reaction or possible anaphylaxis is likely to occur quickly and to be severe. Be sure that you document all medications correctly; include the name of the medication, dose and route, time administered, and patient response. Also be aware that the patient has a right to know about any medications that have been prescribed and has the right to refuse any medication. The other important safety precautions that you must follow are the seven basic rights of medication administration listed in Table 4-8. Many facilities are implementing bar coding procedures for medication administration that will verify the seven rights. However, such procedures do not eliminate your responsibility or accountability during medication administration. Finally, it is important for you to know whether the medication is a **high-alert medication** that can cause significant patient harm if an error is made or if the medication is used incorrectly.

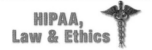
Medication Errors

Health care providers are responsible for knowing about the medications they are giving, including normal dose, proper administration, and possible side effects. They must follow the policies and procedures that were established to facilitate safe medication administration. Health care providers are likewise responsible for reporting any errors made during medication administration. Reporting errors is important because the patient must receive appropriate follow-up care and because the reason for the error must be investigated. For example, was the order and medication sheet legible? Did the error involve a look-alike or soundalike medication? Was the error a calculation error? Was the problem within the system, such as a computer issue in the accessing of electronic records?

Checkpoint Questions 4-5

1. What are the advantages and disadvantages of administering medications by the IV route?

_____

_____

2. Name the seven rights of medication administration.

_____

_____

 Before you continue to the chapter summary, answer the previous Checkpoint Questions and complete the Common IV Medications activity under Chapter 4 on the student CD.

Chapter Summary

- There are three categories of IV fluids: isotonic, hypertonic, and hypotonic. Isotonic solutions have the same osmolarity that serum does. Hypertonic solutions have an osmolarity that is higher than that of serum, and hypotonic solutions have an osmolarity that is lower than that of serum.

- IV solutions contain different concentrations of sodium chloride, dextrose, a combination of dextrose and sodium chloride, electrolytes, or plasma expanders. The choice of IV solution is based on patient requirements for maintenance, replacement, or plasma expansion.

- Patients receive blood and blood products intravenously to restore circulating blood volume, to improve the ability of the blood to carry oxygen, and to replace components the body is lacking. The blood donor and the recipient must be carefully matched for ABO and Rh compatibility to prevent hemolytic transfusion reaction.

- Parenteral nutrition is used to supply nutrients to patients who cannot eat or tolerate nutrients via the gastrointestinal tract. Peripheral parenteral nutrition provides minimal calories and proteins for a short time because highly concentrated dextrose solutions cannot be infused peripherally. Total parenteral nutrition is administered through a central vein, will restore or maintain a patient's nutritional status, and may be used for long-term nutritional support.

- Heparin prevents blood clots from expanding and new clots from forming. Patients on heparin drips must be closely monitored for signs of bleeding and hemorrhage.

- IV insulin infusions are used to decrease the amount of glucose in patients who are in diabetic ketoacidosis. The blood glucose level of these patients must be carefully monitored, and these patients must be closely observed for signs of hypoglycemia.

- Vitamins and electrolytes are administered intravenously to replace patient losses. They are frequently added to TPN solutions, but they may also be given individually, based on patient need.

- Compatibility of IV solution components is crucial to therapeutic response. Compatibility may be affected by the following factors: order of mixing, drug concentration, time, temperature, light exposure, and pH. Incompatibility causes the loss of effects of the medication and may be physical, chemical, or therapeutic.

- To prevent compatibility problems, IV components should be reconstituted correctly, infused with the correct solution, changed every 24 hours, and discarded if the solution changes color or forms a precipitate.

- Medications are introduced directly into the bloodstream so that therapeutic levels are reached quickly and lower doses are needed. Dosages can be easily adjusted based on patient response.

- Two common methods of classifying medications are the generic/trade name classification and the functional or therapeutic classification, which is based on the medication's clinical indication, the body system affected, and the pharmacology of the medication.

- Patient safety is a primary concern during the administration of any medication. Orders must be reviewed by a pharmacist and verified by a health care professional prior to administration. Health care providers administering medication must ensure that they are giving the right medication to the right patient, at the right time, in the right dose, and by the right route. In addition, they must thoroughly document all medication administration, including date and time, route, and patient response.

Matching

_____ **1.** hemolytic reaction

_____ **2.** Rh system

_____ **3.** osmolarity

_____ **4.** hypertonic solution

_____ **5.** ABO system

_____ **6.** incompatibility

_____ **7.** parenteral nutrition

_____ **8.** isotonic solution

_____ **9.** extravasation

_____ **10.** hypotonic solution

a. solution that draws fluids from cells and tissues

b. a chemical, physical, or therapeutic change that occurs when two or more medication or solutions are mixed

c. the inadvertent infiltration of necrotizing solutions or medications into surrounding tissue

d. blood transfusion reaction caused by a donor/recipient incompatibility

e. solution that moves across the cell membrane into surrounding cells and tissues

f. inherited antigens found on the surface of red blood cells; the second most important system for determining donor/recipient compatibility

g. solution that does not affect the fluid balance of the surrounding cells or tissues

h. concentration of a solution; determines the direction of fluid shift between the extracellular and intracellular compartments

i. IV infusion of nutrients, including amino acids, dextrose, fat, electrolytes, vitamins, and trace elements

j. blood grouping system based on antigens present on red blood cells and antibodies in the serum; the most important system for determining donor/recipient compatibility

True/False

T   F   **11.** Patients with congestive heart disease must be monitored for fluid overload when receiving a sodium chloride IV solution.

T   F   **12.** Plasma expanders act to expand the intracellular space.

T   F   **13.** Blood and blood products are the body's main transport for oxygen, nutrients, and hormones.

T   F   **14.** Total parenteral nutrition can be used for long-term nutritional support.

T   F   **15.** Incompatibility does not cause the loss of therapeutic effects of a medication or solution.

Multiple Choice

16. Which type of IV solution causes no movement of fluids into or out of the intravascular space?
    a. sodium chloride
    b. hypertonic
    c. isotonic
    d. hypotonic

17. Hypertonic solutions have an osmolarity that is
    a. higher than that of serum.
    b. lower than that of serum.
    c. the same as that of serum.
    d. none of the above

18. Which of the following describes the effect of hypotonic solutions on fluid movement?
    a. Fluid shifts out of the cells into the intravascular space.
    b. Fluid is not affected.
    c. Circulatory overload takes place.
    d. Fluid shifts into the cells from the intravascular space.

19. Which of the following can cause a hemolytic reaction?
    a. ABO incompatibility
    b. a normal saline infusion
    c. Rh incompatibility
    d. both a and c

20. Which of these solutions will restore and maintain nutritional status for patients?
    a. peripheral parenteral nutrition
    b. total parenteral nutrition
    c. D5 NS
    d. Ringer's solution

21. Which of these IV additives can cause hemorrhage or bleeding?
    a. insulin
    b. potassium
    c. heparin
    d. morphine

22. Which of these factors affects drug compatibility?
    a. order in which drugs are mixed
    b. time and temperature
    c. light and pH
    d. all of the above

23. Which of the following is an advantage of IV medication administration?
    a. possibility of drug incompatibility
    b. rapid drug actions and therapeutic response
    c. extravasation
    d. loss of therapeutic action

24. Which of the following classifications of medications is used to treat cancer?
    a. anti-infectives
    b. antifungals
    c. chemotherapeutic agents
    d. analgesics

25. Which of the following rights are included in the seven basic rights of medication administration?
    a. right drug, right patient, right time, right route, and right dose
    b. right drug, right patient, right doctor, right route, and right dose
    c. right drug, right room, right time, right route, and right dose
    d. right drug, right patient, right date, right route, and right dose

What Should You Do? (Critical Thinking/Application)

1. You are preparing to give a 45-year-old male patient an IV antibiotic. You ask him if he has any allergies. He says that he thinks so; he cannot remember what the medication is but he does know it makes him very sick. What should you do?

   _____

   _____

   _____

2. When checking the IV of your 55-year-old female patient, you notice that the date on the bag's label is 2 days old and that the solution appears cloudy. About 300 mL remains in the bag. The IV is running at a keep-open rate of 15 mL/hour via an infusion pump, so the infusion will last through your shift. What should you do?

   _____

   _____

   _____

Get Connected

Visit the McGraw-Hill Higher Education website for *Intravenous Therapy for Health Care Personnel* at **www.mhhe.com/healthcareskills** to complete the following activity.

1. You have been asked to help write the policy for the use of high-alert medications at your facility. Use the Internet to visit the websites of at least three agencies or facilities to gather your information; then write a policy that includes a list of medications considered to be high-alert and instructions on how they are to be handled in order to prevent medication errors.

Using the Student CD

Now that you have completed the material in Chapter 4, return to the student CD and complete any chapter activities you have not yet done. Practice your terminology with the Key Term Concentration game. Review the chapter material with the Spin the Wheel game. Take the final chapter test, complete the troubleshooting question, and e-mail or print your results to document your proficiency for this chapter.

Preparation and Patient Communication

5

Chapter Outline

   I. Introduction

  II. Preparation for the IV Infusion
- **a.** Physician's Orders
- **b.** Patient Preparation
    - **i.** Psychological Preparation
    - **ii.** Physical Preparation

 III. Patient Identification and Screening
- **a.** Screening before an IV Infusion
- **b.** Screening and Monitoring during IV Administration

 IV. Site Selection for Peripheral IVs
- **a.** Site Selection
- **b.** Peripheral Veins
    - **i.** Dorsal Digital Veins
    - **ii.** Metacarpal Veins
    - **iii.** Cephalic Vein
    - **iv.** Accessory Cephalic Vein
    - **v.** Basilic Vein
    - **vi.** Median Cephalic and Median Basilic Veins
    - **vii.** Median Antebrachial Vein
    - **viii.** Other Sites

  V. Preparation of Supplies and Equipment

 VI. Initiation of Peripheral IV Therapy

VII. Special Populations
- **a.** Geriatric Patients
- **b.** Obese Patients
- **c.** Pediatric Patients
    - **i.** Immobilization
    - **ii.** Venipuncture Sites

Learning Outcomes

- Identify a correctly written order for an IV infusion.
- Prepare the patient psychologically and physically for IV therapy.
- Select and prepare the correct equipment for IV therapy based on the physician's order and the facility policy.

- Demonstrate the process for setting up the IV infusion.
- Describe the anatomical structures and functions of veins utilized as venipuncture sites.
- Identify and select appropriate veins commonly used for venipuncture.
- Aseptically prepare a site for venipuncture.
- Discuss and be able to demonstrate IV therapy techniques for insertion of a peripheral IV and saline or heparin lock.
- Discuss factors to consider when preparing and initiating IVs in geriatric, obese, and pediatric patients.

Key Terms

anesthetic cream
cannulation
EMLA
flash
IV flow sheet
mastectomy

MAR
palpate
rehydration
skin turgor
valves
venipuncture

5-1 Introduction

The ability to obtain IV access is an essential skill in medicine and is performed in a variety of settings, most commonly by paramedics, nurses, and physicians. Other health care professionals, including medical assistants, are now being given IV therapy training so that they will be able to monitor and, in some states, initiate IV therapy. The actual initiation of the IV may appear deceptively simple when performed by an expert; however, it is in fact a difficult skill that demands considerable practice to perfect.

Initiation of IV therapy requires numerous basic preparatory steps. These include:

- Verify the physician's orders
- Gather the equipment
- Introduce yourself to the patient
- Identify the patient
- Provide for patient privacy
- Position the patient
- Wash your hands and put on gloves

As you learned in Chapter 2, the potential for contact with a patient's blood while starting an IV is high, and it increases with the inexperience of the health care professional. Standard Precautions and aseptic technique must be adhered to at all times; for example, the health care professional must wear gloves when starting an IV. If the risk of blood splatter is high, such as with an agitated patient, the health care professional should also wear face and eye protection and a gown. (In trauma situations and in emergency rooms, all health care team members are required to wear gloves, face and eye protection, and gowns.) Once the protective sheath has been removed from the venous access device, the device should immediately be inserted into the patient's vein or disposed of in the appropriate sharps container. Strict compliance with sharps disposal can help prevent inadvertent needlesticks.

This chapter guides you through the preparation of an IV infusion, the physical and psychological preparation of the patient, the selection of the site, and the competencies related to the initiation of the infusion.

Checkpoint Questions 5-1

1. What are the basic preparatory steps for initiating an IV?

   _____

   _____

2. Why is it imperative that Standard Precautions and aseptic technique be adhered to during IV therapy?

   _____

   _____

5-2 Preparation for the IV Infusion

Two important steps that you must follow before starting an IV infusion are (1) obtain and check the physician's order and (2) prepare the patient physically and psychologically for the infusion.

Physician's Orders

Once the physician gives an order for the initiation of IV therapy, you must carry out the procedure in the shortest amount of time possible. Recall from Chapter 1 that a common reason for IV therapy is **rehydration** (fluid replacement). Expediency is essential if fluid replacement is the reason IV therapy was ordered. Continued loss of fluid is a critical condition, and as the patient becomes more severely dehydrated, you will find it more difficult to access peripheral veins.

The patient's medical record should contain a written order for IV therapy, which you must review before initiating the procedure. The order explains the type and amount of fluid to be used and the rate of the infusion. For example, "1000 mL D5W q8h" means "infuse 1000 milliliters of 5% dextrose in water every (over) eight hours." Another example is "500 mL D5W@50 mL per hour." This order means "infuse 5% dextrose in water at a rate of 50 milliliters an hour, and hang a bag that contains 500 milliliters." If the IV order is not clear or is missing any information, check with the ordering practitioner before you proceed. You will also want to determine if the patient is scheduled for any surgical or diagnostic procedures, because this information may dictate the size of the venous access device that you use. If the IV therapy includes an infusion pump, select the proper tubing. If the patient is to receive medication in addition to fluids, use tubing that has an access port. After you have determined the correctness of the order and have gathered all the information, you (or the health care professional who will be starting the IV) should take time to evaluate the patient physically and psychologically and prepare him or her for the procedure.

The physician's order for your patient reads "1000 mL of NSS@125 mL/h."
You are preparing the equipment and supplies for the IV procedure.

What type of fluid will you be infusing?

_____

_____

At what rate will the fluid run, in milliliters per hour?

_____

_____

What is the size of the IV fluid container that you will hang?

_____

_____

Patient Preparation

Before you gather the equipment for an IV infusion, take a few minutes to
talk with the patient. Spending this time now may save you some steps and
time in the long run. Go to the patient and provide for privacy so that you
can speak without interruption. Remember, privacy is a strict requirement of
HIPAA regulations. If the patient is a child, is elderly, or is confused, ask that
a family member remain with the patient to assist with the explanation and
to provide permission for the procedure. Introduce yourself to the patient,
and make sure that you also state your title. Identify the patient by asking
his or her name and checking the identification armband. If the patient
does not have an armband, follow your facility's policy for proper patient
identification. (Recall from Chapter 1 that JCAHO patient safety standards
require two forms of patient identification.) See the accompanying Patient
Education and Communication box for dialogue suggestions.

Patient Education & Communication / Establishing Patient Contact

During your first contact with a patient who will be receiving an IV, introduce yourself and provide an explanation of the procedure. For example,
you might start by saying, "Good morning, Mr. Hanson. I am Hector Stone,
the medical assistant assigned to care for you today. Dr. Rice has ordered
an IV for you. This means that you will be receiving fluids or medications
directly into a vein in your arm. In order to do this, a needle is inserted
through your skin and into your vein. Once I have accessed your vein, the
needle is removed and only a small plastic tube will remain. The device
that contains the fluids or medications will be connected to the tube. Do
you have any questions?" After you have answered all questions to the
patient's satisfaction, you can say, "I will go and gather the equipment
needed, and then come back to get the IV started."

Psychological Preparation

Give the patient a thorough explanation of the IV infusion procedure, including the rationale (why the procedure is being done), what the patient can do to help the procedure run smoothly, what the patient should avoid doing, and roughly how long the IV infusion will be in progress. Also, consider the potential effects of the procedure on the patient's relatives. For example, parents might be concerned by the fact that their child is attached to an IV infusion. Patients and family members may be disturbed by the alarms on the electronic infusion device. Explain what your action will be in the event that an alarm sounds.

Many patients have a fear of needles. Explain to the patient that a needle with a plastic cannula, or tube, is used to penetrate the skin and vein, but once in place, the needle is removed and only the plastic tube (cannula) remains. Do not deceive the patient when he or she asks about pain, but assure the patient that the pain will be short in duration. Explain that although the patient must remain still during the insertion, once the IV is in place and secured, he or she will be able to move about and use the arm.

Allow the patient to express fears and concerns. A few minutes spent validating the patient's feelings and explaining the procedure fully is time well spent. It may encourage the patient to be more cooperative, and the infusion may proceed more smoothly.

Physical Preparation

Make the patient comfortable prior to beginning the IV infusion procedure. Assist the patient to the bathroom, or offer a bedpan. If the patient is wearing street clothes or pajamas, offer a special IV gown, if appropriate. These gowns have snaps or other fasteners on the shoulders so that the gown can be changed without disturbing the IV (Figure 5-1). Always offer to assist the patient with changing into the gown.

Safety and Infection Control

Changing a Gown

Changing a gown on a patient with an IV can present many safety issues, but these problems can be avoided if the patient is wearing an IV-style gown. If the patient is not wearing an IV-style gown, you will have to remove the administration set from the IV pump and thread the line and the fluid container through the sleeve of the soiled gown as well as through the clean gown. During this process, you must hold the tubing and the bag below the insertion site; if you are not careful, you may cause a backflow into the line or may dislodge the cannula. It is *never* appropriate to disconnect the administration set from the venous access device; doing so compromises sterility and may allow air to enter the line.

In addition to cleaning the IV insertion site, which is discussed later in this chapter, you may need to physically prepare the skin surface, usually the back of the hand or the forearm. Preparation may include removal of any hair, because adhesive tape should not be applied over body hair. If you do need to remove hair, you should clip it, not shave it. Shaving could cut the skin, which would create a portal of entry for infection.

Figure 5-1 Patients with IVs can wear special gowns with snaps or buttons in the sleeves that make the process of changing clothes around the IV and tubing easier.

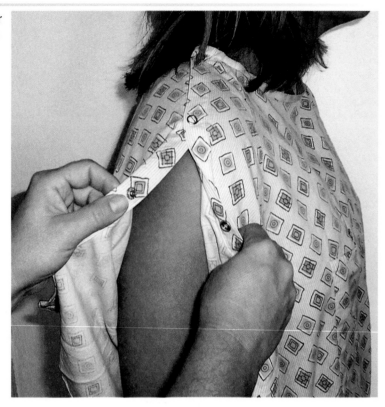

The physician or other health care professional starting the IV may use an anesthetic medication to reduce pain at the insertion site. Either a topical **anesthetic cream** or a local subcutaneous injection of a medication like Xylocaine is common. One brand of topical cream is **EMLA**. This anesthetic reduces the pain of the needlestick. You may be responsible for preparing the injection or for applying the cream. Know your facility's policy regarding the use of anesthetics, and check the manufacturer's directions for the type of anesthetic you are using.

✓ **Checkpoint Questions 5-2**

1. What information is included in the physician's order for an IV infusion?

_____

_____

2. What do you do to prepare the patient psychologically for the IV procedure?

_____

_____

3. What do you do to prepare the patient physically for the IV procedure?

_____

_____

Before you continue to the next section, answer the previous Checkpoint Questions and complete the Preparation for the IV Infusion activity under Chapter 5 on the student CD.

5-3 Patient Identification and Screening

Check the patient's identity before you start an IV procedure and whenever you change the containers of fluid. You cannot be too careful when identifying the patient. Check the patient's identity against the fluid to be administered and against the **IV flow sheet** (also called the IV administration record) or the **MAR** (medication administration record). Perform the *three checks* that are necessary before the administration of any medication: compare the fluid or medication with the physician's order (1) when the fluid or medication is obtained or taken off the shelf, (2) as it is being prepared, and (3) prior to beginning infusion.

If you are initiating an IV infusion, it is your responsibility to follow the *seven rights* explained in Chapter 4: the right medication, the right patient, the right time, the right route, the right dose, the right technique, and the right documentation. In all cases, address the patient by his or her full name, and check the patient's identification number against the IV flow sheet and/or the MAR. In some facilities, you will use a device to scan the patient's identification band and the fluid to be administered; this scanning procedure helps ensure that the proper fluid is given to the correct patient.

Safety and Infection Control

Proper Patient Identification

To be in compliance with JCAHO National Patient Safety Standards, before you perform any IV therapy procedure on a patient, you must properly identify the patient by at least two identifiers (neither of which should be the patient's room number).

Screening before an IV Infusion

The screening procedure that occurs prior to IV infusion includes a clinical screening or examination. It is typically performed by the physician or other licensed practitioner who has ordered the IV infusion. However, if you are the person initiating and monitoring the IV, you may need to provide assistance and to check for certain information. For example, you should check the patient's medical records for allergies and for conditions that could affect the placement of the IV.

Assessing for patient allergies could prevent life-threatening complications. Never proceed with initiation of an IV infusion without checking not only for allergies to the medications that will be administered but also for allergies to latex (used in tourniquets and gloves), tape, alcohol, or povidone iodine (Betadine).

Check the patient's medical records for conditions that could affect placement of the IV. For example, if a patient has cellulitis (infection of the skin), edema, burns, an indwelling fistula for dialysis, sclerosis, or a traumatic injury, you do not want to start an IV distal to (farther away from the body than) this condition. All these problems lead to poor circulation and would consequently interfere with the IV infusion. Another common example, if a patient has had a radical **mastectomy** of the left breast, do not start an IV in the left arm. Circulation may be impaired in the left arm. In most situations, you will not put an IV in an extremity with paralysis or with poor circulation caused by a peripheral vascular disease or related condition such as chronic renal disease or diabetes. If a patient's peripheral circulation is very poor, a central IV line may be ordered.

Screening and Monitoring during IV Administration

Each time you administer a new IV fluid container, you must complete the patient identification procedure again. This rule applies whether you are administering a second primary infusion bag or an IV piggyback of fluids or medications. Always review the patient's medical record, and note any changes that may have occurred. In most cases, you should check the physician's order directly to ensure accuracy. Assess the patient again, both physically and psychologically, and take time to address any questions or concerns.

Monitor the IV therapy to be sure that the prescribed fluid will be delivered over the stated duration. Keep a record of all fluid administered and urine passed. Any degree of fluid imbalance should be reported to the doctor. Regularly record the patient's temperature, blood pressure, pulse, and respiratory rate throughout the procedure. Changes in these conditions could present a warning of impending fluid overload. Fluid overload, or hypervolemia, is a medical condition in which the body has too much fluid. This complication is discussed in more detail in Chapter 6.

On a regular basis and every time you enter the room of a patient undergoing IV therapy, look carefully at the insertion site as well as the fluid container and infusion pump. See if the appropriate amount of fluid has been infused and if the site is in good condition. Observe the skin area for redness, swelling, and temperature. These are signs of phlebitis and infiltration, which are covered in more detail in Chapter 6. Catching a problem early can lessen the discomfort and complications for your patient. Also, look for wetness around the infusion site as well as around and under the extremity. Moisture means that the access device has become dislodged or disconnected, or it may be occluded (blocked). Immediate action needs to be taken. If necessary, discontinue the IV from that site and initiate a new site so that therapy can continue.

Numerous complications can occur with IV therapy. It is important for you to know and understand what problems can happen and how they can be fixed. Chapter 6 provides a description of common complications and instructions for treatment.

Safety and Infection Control

Preparing IV Medication

Never prepare doses of IV medications for more than one patient at a time. Complete the procedure for each patient individually. This will prevent you from inadvertently attaching the wrong piggyback container to a patient's IV. Administration of the wrong medication is a serious error. If a patient is allergic to the incorrect medication, which frequently occurs with antibiotics, a life-threatening situation could occur.

1. You are instructed to initiate an IV on a patient. The patient is unresponsive. Explain the process you will use to identify the patient.

_____

_____

2. List in order of importance the items that you would check prior to initiating IV therapy.

_____

_____

3. Several of your patients are to receive intermittent IV medication. What steps do you take to ensure that you do not make any administration errors?

_____

_____

 Before you continue to the next section, answer the previous Checkpoint Questions and complete the Patient Identification and Screening activity under Chapter 5 on the student CD.

5-4 Site Selection for Peripheral IVs

To select the best peripheral vein for an IV insertion, you must consider several factors about the process and about the patient. In addition, you need a basic understanding of how veins work and where the most common veins are located.

Site Selection

Generally, you will start a peripheral IV at the most distal site (the site farthest away from the body) that is available and appropriate for the situation. This allows **cannulation** (the act of inserting an IV access device into a vein) of a more proximal site (a site closer to the body) if your initial attempt fails. If you first puncture a proximal vein and then try to start an IV distal to that site, fluid may leak from the injured proximal vessel. In circumstances in which the veins of the patient's upper extremities are inaccessible, the veins of the dorsum of the foot or the saphenous vein of the lower leg are sometimes used. See Table 5-1 for some rules on site selection and the preferred order of sites in the upper and lower extremities.

Different situations merit the use of different sites. For example, the preferred sites in emergency care are the veins of the forearm, followed by the median cubital vein that crosses the antecubital fossa. In trauma patients, the first choice is often to go directly to the median cubital vein because it will accommodate a large-bore IV and because it is generally easy to catheterize. In infants and children, a vein in the scalp may be utilized. In newborns, an umbilical vessel is used. In circumstances in which no peripheral IV access is possible, a central IV is started.

TABLE 5-1   Factors in Site Selection for Peripheral IVs

General rules for site selection	Start distally (away from the center of the body) and work proximally (toward the center of the body).
	Avoid the patient's dominant hand, if possible, so the patient can engage in self care when necessary.
Specific rules for site selection	Choose peripheral veins that are straight, large, bifurcated, easily accessible, and surrounded by healthy subcutaneous tissue.
	Make your first attempt in the largest, most prominent vein you can find. It is sometimes easier to feel a vein than to see it.
Upper extremity sites in order of preference	1. Dorsal surface of the hand (dorsal digital, dorsal metacarpal, or dorsal venous network)
	2. Superficial radial and ulnar veins on the forearm (median antebrachial or accessory cephalic)
	3. Cephalic vein located on the radial border of the forearm
	4. Basilic vein on the ulnar portion of the forearm
Lower extremity sites in order of preference	1. Dorsal surface of the foot
	2. Saphenous vein of the ankle

Peripheral Veins

Veins are similar to arteries but because they transport blood at a lower pressure, they are not as strong as arteries. Like arteries, veins have three layers: an outer layer of tissue, a layer of muscle in the middle, and a smooth inner layer of epithelial cells. However, the layers in veins are thinner than in arteries because they contain less tissue (Figure 5-2).

Veins receive blood from the capillaries after the exchange of oxygen and carbon dioxide has taken place. Therefore, the veins transport waste-rich

Figure 5-2 Arteries and veins both have three layers; however, veins are used for IV therapy because they have less pressure and because they transport blood and fluid back to the heart for circulation.

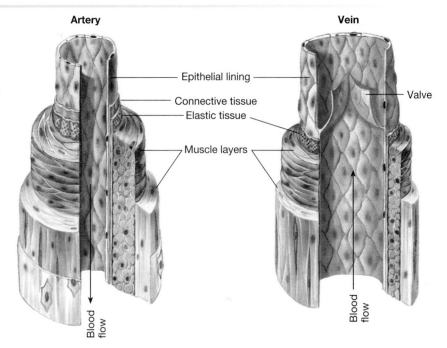

Artery   Vein

Epithelial lining

Connective tissue
Elastic tissue

Valve

Muscle layers

Blood flow

Blood flow

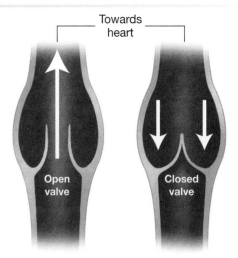

Figure 5-3 Veins have valves that keep the blood flowing toward the heart and against the force of gravity.

Towards heart

Open valve

Closed valve

blood back to the lungs and heart. It is important that the waste-rich blood keeps moving in the proper direction and not be allowed to flow backward. **Valves** located inside the veins prevent this backflow. The valves are like gates that allow traffic to move in only one direction. The vein valves are necessary to keep blood flowing toward the heart, but they are also necessary to allow blood to flow against the force of gravity (Figure 5-3).

It is important that you access the vein far enough from the valve that the end of the catheter does not lay within the valve. If it did, the flow through the catheter could be occluded whenever the valve closes. In general, find a vein section that looks straight. Choose a vein that has a firm, round appearance or feel when palpated. Avoid areas where the vein crosses over joints. An IV in the wrist joint, which contains the radial nerve as well as the tendon that controls the thumb, can cause problems if the cannula is placed too close to these areas. Avoid these problems by moving the insertion site proximally along the vein.

If possible, avoid areas where cannulation or **venipuncture** has previously taken place. Repeated puncture of the vein wall can be painful for a patient. Obtaining a patent cannula is a bonus in any patient who has had multiple venipunctures, which is why health care professionals often use the antecubital veins as a last resort or in emergency situations.

Antecubital veins are easy veins to see as well as to **palpate** (feel). They are also easy to access, but their use as an IV site can be problematic. To prevent the vein from occluding, the patient must keep that arm straight. You will need to use an arm board on the patient, which can be cumbersome and uncomfortable. The following sections and Figures 5-4 and 5-5 provide information about specific vein locations and when they are used.

Safety and Infection Control

Always Use Aseptic Technique

The IV procedure requires an aseptic technique as well as appropriate measures to reduce the risk of contamination. These measures must be upheld throughout the procedure, from setup and priming of the IV, through the initiation of venous access, while fluids are being infused, to the discontinuing of the therapy. Aseptic technique *must* be maintained at all times.

Figure 5-4 Major veins in the hand.

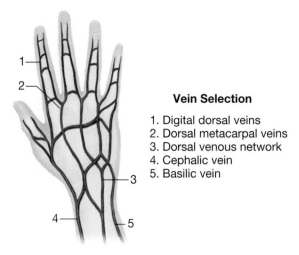

Vein Selection

1. Digital dorsal veins
2. Dorsal metacarpal veins
3. Dorsal venous network
4. Cephalic vein
5. Basilic vein

Digital Dorsal Veins

Dorsal digital veins flow along the lateral portion of fingers and are joined to each other by communicating branches. They can accommodate a small-gauge IV catheter (22 or 24 gauge). An IV that is started here will need to be properly supported, because the bending of the finger can reduce or stop the flow of the infusion. Use a tongue blade or hand board to keep the patient's hand or fingers in place and stable. Although dorsal digital veins are not a primary site choice because of their small size, their location makes them very accessible. The metacarpal bones of the finger serve as a splint for the cannula.

Figure 5-5 Major veins in the arm.

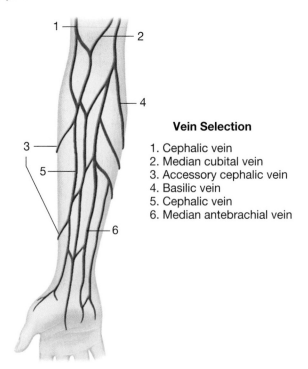

Vein Selection

1. Cephalic vein
2. Median cubital vein
3. Accessory cephalic vein
4. Basilic vein
5. Cephalic vein
6. Median antebrachial vein

Dorsal Metacarpal Veins

Metacarpal veins are formed by the union of digital veins in the dorsal venous area. These veins are a good first choice for IV initiation because they are the most distal site on the extremity. An IV infusion in the metacarpal veins must be properly supported to prevent movement of the IV catheter.

Cephalic Vein

The cephalic vein flows upward along the radial border of the forearm, producing branches to both surfaces of the forearm. Because of their size and location, the branches of the cephalic vein provide excellent sites for IV infusion and can readily accommodate large-gauge IV catheters. The cephalic vein is one of the best veins available for an IV. It tends to be large, and the forearm provides a natural splint.

Accessory Cephalic Vein

The accessory cephalic vein originates from either a plexus on the back of the forearm or the dorsal venous network. It branches off from the cephalic vein just above the wrist and flows back into the main cephalic vein at a higher point. The accessory cephalic vein also can accommodate large-gauge IV catheters. Keep this vein in mind when you move up the patient's forearm in search of acceptable IV site locations.

Basilic Vein

The basilic vein originates in the ulnar portion of the dorsal venous network and ascends along the ulnar portion of the forearm. It curves toward the anterior surface of the arm just below the elbow and meets with the median cubital vein below the elbow. The basilic vein is available for venipuncture above the antecubital fossa (crease on the inner arm) in the upper arm region. The basilic vein is hidden along the ulnar border of the hand and forearm, so it is often overlooked. The vein is fairly large, although it does tend to roll and has numerous valves.

Median Cephalic and Median Basilic Veins

The median cephalic and median basilic veins are located in the antecubital fossa. These two veins should be considered only as a last resort site for blood draws. Neither vein is a favorable site for prolonged infusions.

Median Antebrachial Vein

The median antebrachial vein arises from the venous plexus on the hand and extends along the ulnar side on the anterior surface of the forearm. It empties into the basilic vein or median cubital vein. It is not always easily seen.

Other Sites

Other, less common sites may be used for peripheral IV therapy. These sites most likely will require the expertise of a physician or other licensed practitioner. Veins in the legs and feet, except for the saphenous vein in the ankle and lower leg, are usually not utilized. Small veins on the ventral surface of the wrist or a larger one on the inner aspect of the wrist, proximal to the thumb, may be used, but these locations are not ideal because the ventral surface of the wrist also contains arteries. If these veins are chosen, the most appropriate venous access device is the wing-tipped (butterfly) needle. IV therapy on infants and very young children often utilizes scalp veins. In these situations, the vein is cannulated with a scalp vein needle, which has a small gauge and is usually about 5/8 in. in length. Scalp vein needles have wings to provide a stable grip during insertion.

Checkpoint Questions 5-4

1. List, in order of preference, IV sites in the hand and arm.

_____

_____

2. Why is it not a good idea to use veins in the patient's antecubital fossa (crease of the elbow) for a continuous IV infusion?

_____

_____

Before you continue to the next section, answer the previous Checkpoint Questions and complete the Site Selection for Peripheral IVs activity under Chapter 5 on the student CD.

5-5 Preparation of Supplies and Equipment

Before you can initiate an IV infusion, you must gather and prepare the necessary supplies and equipment (Figure 5-6). The following items are needed:

- An intravenous cannula of the appropriate size
- A fluid administration set

Figure 5-6 Equipment needed to initiate an IV site is pictured here.

A. Tourniquet
B. Two venous access devices
C. 2 X 2 gauze
D. Alcohol prep pad
E. Extension tubing
F. PRN cap
G. Tape strips
H. Semitransparent dressing
I. Needleless access tip for saline syringe
J. Saline flush
K. Gloves

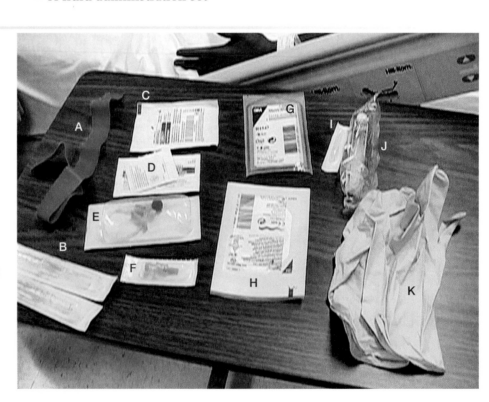

- The prescribed fluid
- The MAR and/or the IV flow sheet or record (Figure 5-7)
- The vital signs graphic sheet or flow chart
- Cannulation and site supplies

Figure 5-7 An IV flow sheet is used to maintain a record during intravenous therapy.

IV Flow Sheet

Solutions	Time	By

Device _____ Site _____

Date/Time Inserted _____

Administered by _____

New Site _____

Device _____ Date/Time _____

Administered by _____

Tubing Labeled/Signature

7-3 _____

3-11 _____

11-7 _____

Date/Time		Fluid Level	Rate mL/HR	GTT/ MIN.	T	P	R	BP	Site CK.Q Hr.	Secondary Sol/Thrpy	Action/Comment	IN
	12 AM											
	1 AM											
	2 AM											
	3 AM											
	4 AM											
	5 AM											
	6 AM											
	7 AM											
											11-7 IV Intake	
	8 AM											
	9 AM											
	10 AM											
	11 AM											
	12 PM											
	1 PM											
	2 PM											
	3 PM											
											7-3 IV Intake	
	4 PM											
	5 PM											
	6 PM											
	7 PM											
	8 PM											
	9 PM											
	10 PM											
	11 PM											
											3-11 IV Intake	

Heparin Lock = HL

Site Key:
Y   =   Intact
* S   =   Swollen
* W   =   Wet/Soiled
* R   =   Red
* Action Key Site Key = Narrative Note

Action Key:
* D/C   =   Discounted RX
* W/C   =   Warm Compresses
* I/C   =   Ice Compresses
* DSC   =   Dressing Change
* R/S   =   IV Restart
* T/C   =   Tubing Change

24 HR. Total _____

Resident Name:		Room #	Physician:	Medical Rec. #

Automated Laser Forms by [adl] Data Systems, Inc. (914) 591-1800   IV_Flow.FRP   SBG 1/97

The type and size of the intravenous cannula that you select is based on the information obtained when you evaluated the patient and on the physician's order. You should have a minimum of two cannula available for the procedure. If you are preparing the supplies and equipment for the health care professional who will be initiating the IV, provide a variety of cannula for selection during the procedure. The patient's age and medical status and the location of viable veins will assist you in determining the appropriate device. Recall what you learned in Chapter 3: to lessen irritation to the vein, use the shortest, smallest gauge that will do the job. Also remember to use a larger cannula if the patient faces the possibility of a blood transfusion in the future.

If an infusion pump is to be used, select an administration set that is compatible with the pump. Always check the prescribed IV fluid against the original physician's order when you initiate an IV. However, once you have started the IV, the appropriate information is recorded on the IV flow sheet or MAR. Take and record the patient's vital signs right before or after the IV is initiated.

The cannulation and site dressing supplies that you will assemble are based on the policy of the facility. Some facilities use prepackaged kits from the manufacturer (Figure 5-8). Typical supplies include

- Disposable sheet
- Alcohol prep pad
- Povidone-iodine (Betadine) or other antiseptic swab such as Chlorhexidine
- Tourniquet
- 4 pieces of tape (preferably paper tape or easy-to-remove tape), precut to approximately 4 in. (10 cm) in length and taped conveniently to the table or stretcher
- Disposable gloves
- Gauze (several pieces of 4 × 4 or 2 × 2)
- Antibiotic ointment or film barrier (depending on facility guidelines)
- Time strip for IV fluid bag

Figure 5-8 Cannulation and site supplies in a single IV start kit sometimes come with or without the venous access device from the manufacturer. The contents of this kit did not include the venous access device(s).

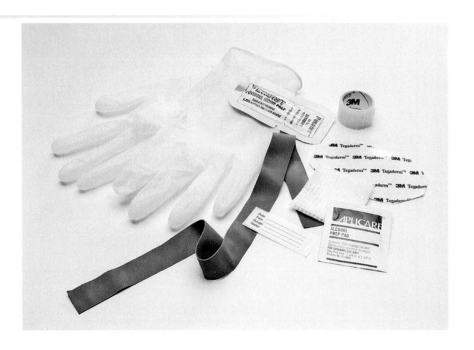

Start by washing your hands. Then select the type of drip chamber you will use based on your evaluation of the patient. Recall from Chapter 3 that the drip chamber will be either microdrip or macrodrip. Uncoil the tubing without letting the ends of the tubing become contaminated by hitting the floor or other surface. Close the flow regulator (by rolling the wheel away from the end you will attach to the fluid bag). Remove the protective covering from the port of the fluid bag and the protective covering from the spike of the administration set. Insert the spike of the administration set into the port of the fluid bag with a quick twist. Do this carefully. Do not puncture yourself or contaminate the puncture spike.

Hold the fluid bag higher than the drip chamber of the administration set. Squeeze the drip chamber once or twice to start the flow. Fill the drip chamber to the marker line, which is approximately one-third full. If you accidentally overfill the chamber, lower the bag below the level of the drip chamber and squeeze some fluid back into the fluid bag. Open the flow regulator and allow the fluid to flush *all* the air from the tubing. Let it run into a trashcan or even the (now empty) wrapper that the fluid bag came in. You may need to loosen or remove the cap at the end of the tubing to get the fluid to flow, although most sets now allow flow without removal. Take care not to let the tip of the administration set become contaminated. Depending on the type of administration set, you may need to invert the inline filter or the mechanism that is inserted into the infusion pump for it to fill properly. Check the manufacturer's directions. Remember, *all* air must be removed, or purged, from the line. Turn off the flow and place the sterile cap back on the end of the administration set (if you had to remove it). Place this end of the IV tubing with the cap loosely in place nearby so that when you initiate the IV, you can reach it quickly and easily in order to attach it to the IV access device.

If you are using an infusion pump, you must program the infusion parameters. You may need to enter the total volume to be infused or the amount of fluid in the bag you are hanging and the rate ordered by the physician. For example, if you have a 1000 mL bag of fluid that is to run at 100 mL an hour, these are the two numbers you will enter. Different brands of pumps have different programming requirements. Always check the manufacturer's instructions. In some facilities, the manufacturer or the facility provides in-service training to teach health care workers about equipment such as infusion pumps. This equipment and its technology change frequently, so make sure you are up-to-date.

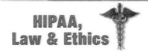

HIPAA, Law & Ethics

Scope of Practice

IV supplies and equipment are updated frequently. It is your responsibility to be familiar with the equipment and supplies you use and monitor during IV therapy. You must work within your scope of practice legally and ethically. Do not use equipment that you are unfamiliar with or unable to operate. If necessary, ask for assistance, because improper use of equipment could lead to an error and possible harm to the patient.

Now that the equipment is gathered and ready, take the IV cannulation and dressing supplies and the primed IV fluid and infusion pump to the patient's bedside. Let the patient know that the IV is going to be initiated.

Provide for privacy, and assist the patient to a comfortable position. Raise the bed to a comfortable working height. Wash your hands or use a hand sanitizer. It is now time to initiate the IV.

Checkpoint Questions 5-5

1. List the supplies that you will gather and prepare before you initiate a peripheral IV.

_____

_____

2. Name at least two ways that you can prevent the spread of infection during the preparation of equipment and supplies.

_____

_____

Before you continue to the next section, answer the previous Checkpoint Questions and complete the Preparation of Supplies and Equipment activity under Chapter 5 on the student CD.

5-6 Initiation of Peripheral IV Therapy

Starting an IV is an art form that is learned through experience, and your ability improves after you have performed many IVs. IV therapy courses provide you with the theory and skills that you need before you begin obtaining the experience. Some patients have veins that are easily accessed, but many patients prove difficult because of their age, physical condition, or level of hydration. Even health care professionals with many years of experience will occasionally encounter a situation in which they are unable to successfully cannulate a vein. Never be reluctant to ask for assistance. Seeking help prevents undue discomfort for your patient and personal frustration for you. As you gain experience, you will be able to assess your own ability and will know when it is appropriate to go it alone or to ask for assistance.

Begin with a vein assessment by examining the veins on the patient's nondominant arm. Apply a tourniquet high on the upper arm (Figure 5-9). The tourniquet should be tight enough to visibly indent the skin but not cause the patient discomfort. To maximize venous engorgement, ask the patient to make a fist several times and to keep the arm lowered. Select the appropriate vein, and palpate it gently to assess its elasticity and rebound filling. If you cannot easily see a suitable vein, you can sometimes feel one by palpating the arm with your fingers (not your thumb, because it is less sensitive than the fingers). The vein will feel like an elastic tube that "gives" under pressure. Apply enough pressure to impede venous flow but do not impinge on arterial flow.

If you are unable to locate a suitable vein, you may try dilating the veins by tapping on them, that is, by gently "slapping" them with the pads of two or three fingers. Tapping lightly over a vein will elicit a mechanical reflex dilation of the vascular walls. Take care to tap lightly to avoid reflex vasoconstriction from pain. If you still cannot find any veins, you may find it helpful to cover the arm in a warm, moist compress to help with peripheral vasodilation. *Do not tap on the vein of a patient who is receiving chemotherapy or anticoagulants. The recommendation of the Infusion Nurses Society is that an inflated blood pressure cuff be used instead of a tourniquet to distend the vein. It is also permissible to use warm compresses and massage the vein distally from the cuff or tourniquet.* If, after a meticulous search, you cannot find an appropriate vein, release the tourniquet from above the elbow and place it around the patient's forearm; search in the distal forearm, wrist, and hand. If you still do not find a suitable vein, move to the other arm. Be careful to stay away from arteries, which are pulsating. Also, avoid leaving the tourniquet on for a period greater than 2 minutes at any one site; doing so can be painful for the patient. Sometimes an application of nitroglycerin ointment (0.4% for children and 2% for adults) can be used to facilitate venous dilation. Be sure to check your facility's policy on use of nitro ointment.

Prepare the tape by opening the package or tearing appropriate size strips and placing on a clean location, and then don disposable (nonlatex) gloves. Reapply the tourniquet 4 to 6 inches above the insertion site. Clean the entry site carefully with the alcohol (70% isopropyl) prep pad (Figure 5-10). Apply in a circular motion, moving from the center out, with friction, for at least 30 seconds (Figure 5-11). Allow the area to dry. Then use the povidone-iodine (Betadine) or other antiseptic solution in the same manner, starting with the entry site and extending outward about 2 inches. If the patient is allergic to iodine, just use the isopropyl alcohol or other antiseptic solution. Follow the rules for your facility. Wait until the solution is dry before starting cannulation. Do not fan the area or blow on it to speed drying; those actions could contaminate the site.

Stabilize the vein by using your nondominant hand to apply traction to the skin below the insertion site (Figure 5-12). This traction will help prevent the vein from rolling (moving around freely under the skin). Traction also facilitates cannulation by increasing surface tension and reducing the amount of pressure required to penetrate the skin. Many people use their thumb to apply this traction. Pull the skin distally toward the wrist in the opposite direction that the needle will be advancing. Be careful not to press too hard, which will compress blood flow in the vein and cause the vein to collapse.

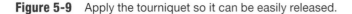

Figure 5-9 Apply the tourniquet so it can be easily released.

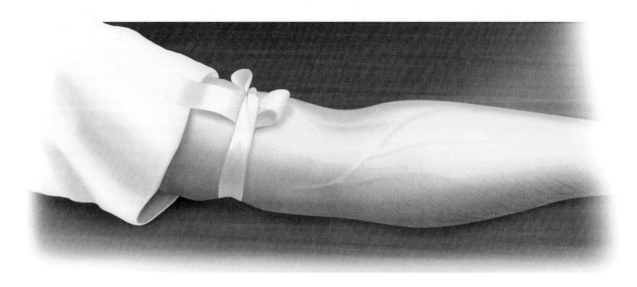

Figure 5-10   Clean the site using a facility approved solution such as alcohol, povidone iodine, or other antiseptic.

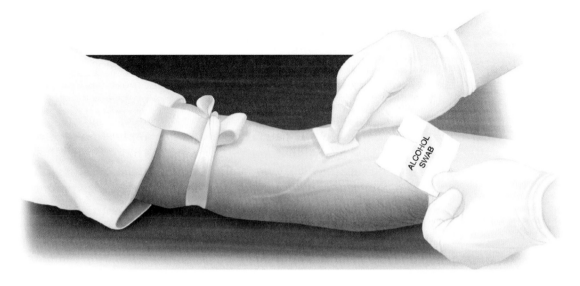

Figure 5-11   Use a circular motion from the center of the site to clean the area that will be cannulated for IV therapy.

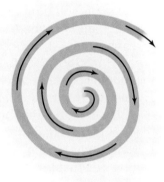

Figure 5-12   Pull the skin in the opposite direction that the needle will be advancing, but do not press too hard.

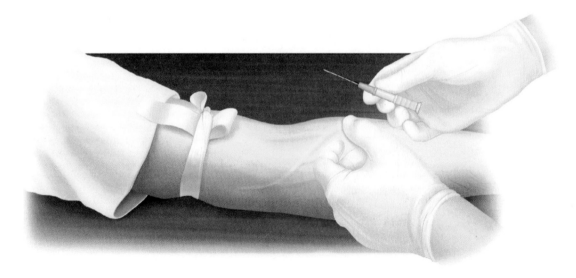

Figure 5-13 With the needle bevel up, use a short, quick motion to pierce the skin but avoid penetrating the vein.

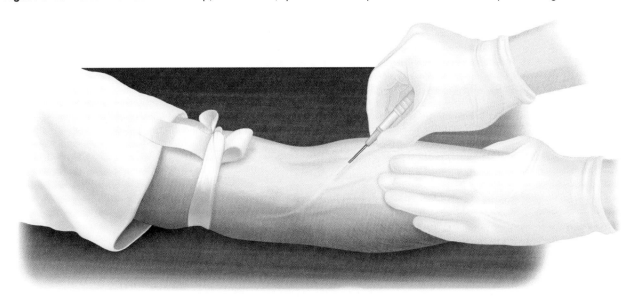

Hold the catheter in your dominant hand. With the bevel up, enter the skin at about a 45-degree angle and in the direction of the vein. Use a quick, short, jabbing motion to pierce the skin until you meet resistance, but avoid penetrating the vein (Figure 5-13). Next, lower the needle angle to nearly parallel to the skin and pierce the vein. You should feel it pop. Advance the catheter to enter the vein until you see blood, or **flash,** in the flash chamber of the catheter. Tilt the needle slightly backward and advance it a bit further to ensure that it is in the vein.

If you are unsuccessful in entering the vein and you do not see a flash of blood, slowly withdraw the catheter without pulling it all the way out, and carefully watch for the flash to occur. If you are still not within the vein, advance it again in a second attempt to enter the vein. Each time that you withdraw, always stop before pulling the needle all the way out; you want to avoid repeating the painful initial skin puncture. If, after one or two manipulations, you have not successfully entered the vein, then release the tourniquet, place a gauze pad over the skin puncture site, withdraw the catheter, tape down the gauze, and discard the device. With a new cannula, try again in the other arm or at a more proximal site. *If your second attempt is unsuccessful, it is best to ask for assistance from someone with more IV experience.* Follow facility policy for the number of repeated attempts permitted.

After you have successfully entered the vein, advance the plastic catheter (which is over the needle) into the vein while leaving the needle stationary (Figure 5-14). The hub of the catheter should be touching the skin puncture site, and the plastic catheter should slide forward easily. Do not force it! Release the tourniquet (Figure 5-15).

Apply gentle pressure over the vein just proximal to the entry site to prevent blood flow. Remove the needle from within the plastic catheter. Dispose of the needle in an appropriate sharps container. *Never reinsert the needle into the plastic catheter while it is in the patient's arm! Reinserting the*

Figure 5-14 After the needle has entered the vein, advance the plastic catheter while leaving the needle in place.

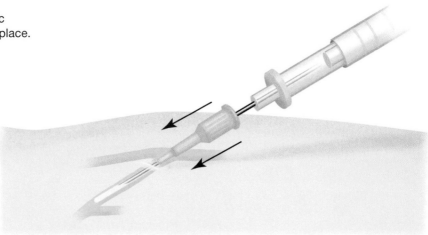

needle can shear off the tip of the plastic catheter, causing an embolus. Remove the protective cap from the end of the administration set and connect it to the plastic catheter (Figure 5-16). Adjust the flow rate as necessary.

Tape the catheter in place with the strips of tape and/or a clear dressing. Label the IV site with the date, time, the gauge and length of the catheter, and your initials. Monitor the infusion for proper flow into the vein (in other words, watch for signs of infiltration such as swelling, cool to touch, or pain) (Figure 5-17).

Once the dressing is in place and the infusion is flowing properly, remove all supplies and extra equipment from the patient's room. In most facilities, supplies that are heavily soiled with blood are handled as biohazard waste. Dispose of sharps in a biohazard container. Be sure that the needles are completely within the container to prevent other health care workers from injury the next time the container is used.

Figure 5-15 Release the tourniquet after advancing the plastic catheter.

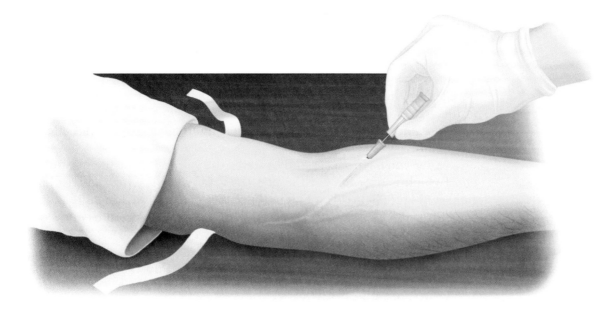

Figure 5-16 Remove the protective cap from the administration set and connect it to the plastic catheter.

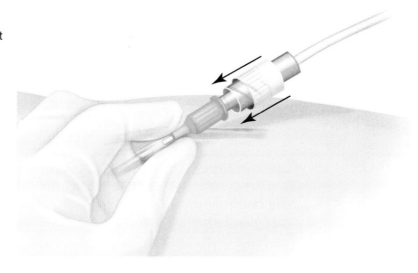

Figure 5-17 Tape the tubing securely, and label the dressing with the date, time, and your initials.

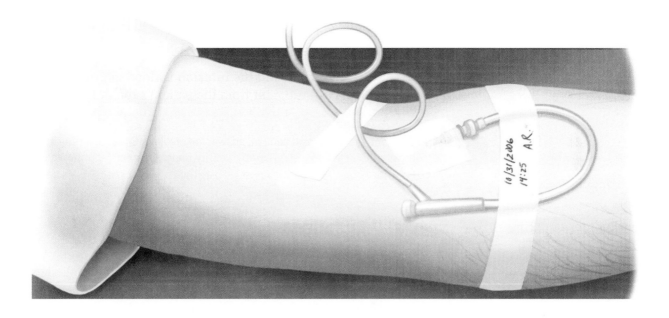

Your final step is to document the procedure. Your documentation should include the following information:

- Insertion site
- Size of cannula
- Type of IV fluid
- Rate of infusion or flush
- Number of attempts
- Patient response
- Signature and title of inserter

For example, your documentation might read as follows: *IV started with 20-gauge angiocath in left forearm on first attempt. Patient tolerated procedure without complaint. 1000 mL of NSS infusing at 100 mL/h. Semitransparent Drsg applied. R. Findley, RN*

Safety and Infection Control

Do Not Reinsert a Venous Access Device

Once a venous access device has been inserted through the skin and the cannulation has been unsuccessful, that needle is contaminated. Using it again could cause a multitude of problems related to infection control, and if the device is a stylet within a plastic cannula, reinserting the stylet could cause shearing of the catheter, which could introduce plastic fragments into the patient's bloodstream.

Checkpoint Questions 5-6

1. How do you prevent the vein from rolling during IV insertion?

   _____

   _____

2. What is the meaning of the term *flash* as it relates to IV initiation?

   _____

   _____

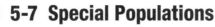

Before you continue to the next section, answer the previous Checkpoint Questions and complete the Initiation of IV Therapy activity under Chapter 5 on the student CD.

5-7 Special Populations

Certain populations of individuals require special consideration when you initiate an IV. These populations are geriatric patients (older adults), obese patients, and pediatric patients (children).

Geriatric Patients

When selecting a vein for IV therapy on a geriatric patient, avoid the back of the hand. This area in an older adult lacks **skin turgor** (elasticity) and has limited subcutaneous tissue, which makes it difficult to cannulate. Limited subcutaneous tissue also makes it difficult to stabilize the cannula after insertion and increases the risk of dislodgment. The skin of the older patient is thinner, and superficial veins tend to be weaker and more prone to infiltration.

You may want to use only hand pressure above the potential IV site rather than a tourniquet to distend the vein. For most elderly patients, this amount of pressure will engorge the vein successfully and eliminate the need for a tourniquet.

Because older patients often suffer from reduced kidney function or chronic disease, they are more prone to fluid overload. The infusion rate and vital signs of these patients must be carefully monitored. Always use a pump to control the infusion rate. Take and record vital signs at least every four hours, perhaps more frequently depending on the patient's condition.

Obese Patients

You may have trouble seeing and palpating a vein suitable for IV cannulation in an obese patient. Overlying tissue may develop collateral circulation, and disease states exacerbated by obesity can impede vein access. Some tips for an easier IV insertion in an obese patient may also help in patients with peripheral edema. Consider the following techniques:

- Warmth encourages vasodilation. Apply warm compresses to the site for 10 to 15 minutes before you attempt cannulation.
- Displace edema and extra tissue. You may need an assistant to help hold extra or edematous tissue out of the way while you insert an IV cannula. Because adipose tissue is often compressible, hold firm finger pressure over a spot at which you are likely to find a vein and try to see or feel one in the depression. Before prepping, make an indentation on the skin with finger pressure, mark the spot with a sterile marker, or have your prepping solution and cannula ready to use quickly.
- Use anatomical landmarks. For example, most people have a superficial vein on the thumb side of the wrist. If your patient wears a wristwatch, which has a mild tourniquet effect, you may see a vein in the indentation left by the watchband. However, because of the risk of nerve injuries and extremely painful venipuncture, use this area only if no other veins are available or if the situation is an emergency.
- Use multiple tourniquets. To distend veins, progress distally from the most proximal joint toward the site.

Pediatric Patients

If the pediatric patient is old enough to understand, explain the IV therapy procedure in appropriate language just before you start. Be honest (do not say, "This won't hurt"). Decide whether the parents should remain with the patient during the procedure. If the parents stay, they should play a comforting role; the parents should not be expected to restrain the child.

Immobilization

Immobilization can be accomplished by either holding or wrapping the infant or child. If holding the child firmly is not sufficient to keep him or her immobile for a procedure, use a wrapping technique. This technique is often needed for children between the ages of 1 and 6. Wrap the child in a sheet or blanket as shown in Figure 5-18. If you are using a limb for IV access, leave it outside the wrapping.

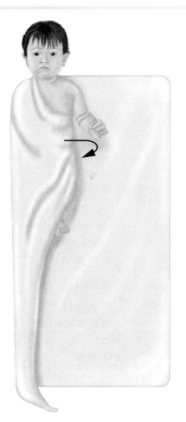
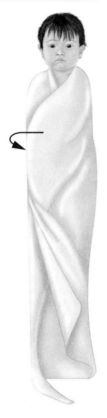
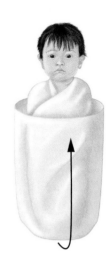

Venipuncture Sites

The preferred sites for IV insertions in pediatric patients are the veins of the upper extremities. The first choices are the forearm veins (e.g., the cephalic vein, the median basilic vein, or the median antecubital vein), but these veins can be difficult to locate in chubby babies. Second-choice sites are the tributaries of the cephalic and basilic veins and the dorsal venous arch. A third option is the small vein on the ventral surface of the wrist or the larger one on the inner aspect of the wrist proximal to the thumb. Scalp veins are an alternative site in infants less than 1 year old. Use a rubber band around the scalp for a tourniquet if necessary. A site of last resort is the saphenous vein, which lies just anterior to the medial malleolus (anklebone). IV access in the scalp or lower extremity of a pediatric patient is usually initiated by a physician. Before accessing a scalp vein, the saphenous vein, or other veins in the lower extremities, check your facility's policy and your state regulations.

Safety and Infection Control

Do Not Recap Needles

Avoid recapping needles, putting catheters back into their sheath, or dropping sharps to the floor (an unfortunate but common practice in trauma situations). The recapping of needles is one of the most common causes of preventable needlestick injuries in health care workers.

1. What precautions should you take when providing IV therapy to a geriatric patient?

_____

_____

2. What techniques can you use when initiating an IV on an obese patient?

_____

_____

 Before you continue to the chapter summary, answer the previous Checkpoint Questions and complete the Special Populations activity under Chapter 5 on the student CD.

Chapter Summary

- A correctly written IV order includes the type, rate, and amount of fluid to be infused.
- Patients must be prepared both psychologically and physically before the initiation of an infusion. The patient is given an explanation of the procedure, the patient's fears are recognized and addressed, and the patient's potential IV site is prepped.
- The basic equipment and supplies needed for IV therapy will vary depending on the policies of the facility. Typical equipment and supplies are the cannula, fluid administration set, prescribed fluid, MAR, physician's order, IV flow sheet, vital signs record, and cannulation and site supplies.
- The correct fluid and appropriate administration set must be used, and the tubing must be aseptically purged prior to IV initiation.
- Veins transport waste-rich blood back to the heart. The valves in the veins keep the blood moving in the proper direction. These valves should be avoided when an IV is started.
- The most common veins used for peripheral IVs are in back of the hand and forearm. Veins on the thumb side of the wrist and in the antecubital space should be avoided.
- Site preparation for IV therapy requires hand hygiene and a cleaning of the site in a circular motion with alcohol, povidone iodine (Betadine), and/or an antiseptic, as recommended by the facility.
- The steps to be followed in the initiation of an IV are (1) stabilize the vein below the insertion site; (2) enter the skin at a 45-degree angle, and then reduce the angle to enter the vein; (3) watch for a flash of blood; (4) ensure that the IV is in the vein; and (5) stabilize the catheter and remove the needle.
- Geriatric, obese, and pediatric patients require special considerations in the initiation of an IV. Patients should always be treated as individuals.

Multiple Choice

1. When selecting an appropriate vein for IV infusion, which of the following factors should you consider?
   a. Veins are deep and large.
   b. Needle is placed near a joint.
   c. Proximal end of the vein is used first.
   d. Vein location allows for mobility.

2. Which of the following is the best action after your first attempt to start an IV and you do not see a flash of blood in the chamber?
   a. Ask the patient to make a fist while you check for blood return in the cannula.
   b. Document the results.
   c. Reattempt to start the IV in another site.
   d. Reuse the cannula and attempt to start at another location.

3. When administering IV therapy to a geriatric patient, which of the following actions should you take?
   a. Use a varicose vein.
   b. Avoid using the dorsal vein because of limited subcutaneous tissue.
   c. Use multiple tourniquets to distend the vein adequately.
   d. Avoid the use of tape.

4. Which of the following factors should you consider when you select an IV site?
   a. Avoid areas that have a round appearance.
   b. Avoid areas where the vein crosses over joints.
   c. Generally use large, protruding veins.
   d. Avoid veins that appear firm when palpated.

5. Which of the following actions should you take in order to become *proficient* in venipuncture techniques?
   a. Practice on an anatomical training arm.
   b. Pass a certification class.
   c. Initiate many IVs on real patients.
   d. Observe an IV team nurse in action.

6. Which of the following statements do you need to remember in order to avoid inadvertently puncturing an artery?
   a. Arteries are frequently damaged during venipuncture.
   b. Arteries and veins are found close together in the antecubital fossa.
   c. Arteries pulsate.
   d. Veins are deep, arteries are superficial.

7. Which of the following actions should you take when you initiate peripheral IV access?
    a. Start with the patient's dominant hand.
    b. Avoid rotating from one extremity to the other.
    c. Start with the most proximal site available.
    d. Avoid routine use of veins in or above the antecubital fossa.

8. Which of the following actions should you take if your initial insertion is not successful?
    a. Remove the cannula tip from the skin and reposition it.
    b. Remove the cannula, properly discard it, and insert a new one at another site.
    c. Reinsert the stylet into the catheter and try again.
    d. Reuse the catheter for a second venipuncture.

9. Your study group is preparing for the IV course final exam. You are discussing venipuncture site preparation. Which of the following statements demonstrates an understanding of the theory?
    a. "The area must be shaved to remove excess hair from the site."
    b. "Clean the area with 70% isopropyl alcohol or other approved antiseptic."
    c. "A back-and-forth motion should be used to clean the area."
    d. "Blot excess antimicrobial solution at the insertion site."

Number the Steps

10. Number the steps of IV cannulation in their proper order (1 to 17).
    _____ release the tourniquet
    _____ tape the IV tubing to the skin
    _____ select the insertion site
    _____ put on gloves
    _____ select the equipment
    _____ insert the cannulation device
    _____ prepare the patient
    _____ dilate and palpate the vein
    _____ prepare the solution set
    _____ review the order for IV access
    _____ withdraw the needle
    _____ document the procedure
    _____ select the cannulation device
    _____ connect the fluid-filled tubing to the hub
    _____ advance the cannulation device
    _____ apply a clear sterile dressing
    _____ prepare the site

Matching

_____ 11. anesthetic cream

_____ 12. cannulation

_____ 13. MAR

_____ 14. flash

_____ 15. IV flow sheet

_____ 16. infiltration

_____ 17. phlebitis

_____ 18. skin turgor

_____ 19. valves

_____ 20. palpate

a. elastic properties of the skin, reflecting the body's fluid status

b. structures within the vein to keep blood flowing toward the heart and against the force of gravity

c. electronic or written record that documents the amount and type of IV fluid

d. medication administration record

e. irritation of the vein caused by mechanical, chemical, or bacterial injury

f. the act of inserting a venous access device into a vein for intravenous therapy

g. to examine by touch; to feel

h. the appearance of blood in a venous access device

i. a solid medication used to reduce pain during venipuncture procedures

j. the leakage of intravenous drugs from the vein into the surrounding tissue

True/False

T   F   **21.** A winged needle is preferred for the transfusion of blood.

T   F   **22.** If you are using an over-the-needle catheter to start an IV on a pediatric patient, gauges of 20 to 26 are the best choices for insertions.

T   F   **23.** Arteries pulsate on palpation.

T   F   **24.** Arteries are commonly used for intravenous therapy.

T   F   **25.** Veins contain valves and carry blood away from the heart.

What Should You Do? (Critical Thinking/Application Questions)

1. Your patient was admitted to the emergency room following an MVA (motor vehicle accident). She has a fractured femur and pelvis. She is responsive but confused. The ER physician has ordered an IV of D5W. As you are removing her clothes, you notice that she is wearing a medic alert tag that identifies her as a diabetic. What action would you take prior to initiating the IV infusion?

_____

_____

_____

2. You are caring for a patient on her day of surgery. She is 60 in. tall and weighs approximately 250 lb. When you inspect the IV site, you find it difficult to determine if the site is edematous or reflects her normal appearance. The area surrounding the IV site is cooler to the touch than is the remainder of her arm. The site is covered with gauze and is taped securely. An infusion pump is being used, and it is not sounding an alarm. What actions would you take to assess the situation?

_____

_____

_____

Get Connected

Visit the McGraw-Hill Higher Education website for *Intravenous Therapy for Health Care Personnel* at **www.mhhe.com/healthcareskills** to complete the following activity.

1. As you learn about IV therapy, you also learn a lot of new terminology. Choose at least five new words from this chapter, and look up their definitions on the medical dictionary found at the website for MedlinePlus.

Using the Student CD

Now that you have completed the material in Chapter 5, return to the student CD and complete any chapter activities you have not yet done. Practice your terminology with the Key Term Concentration game. Review the chapter material with the Spin the Wheel game. Take the final chapter test, complete the troubleshooting question, and e-mail or print your results to document your proficiency for this chapter.

6 Monitoring and Maintaining Intravenous Therapy

Chapter Outline

I. Introduction
II. Labeling
   a. Site Label
   b. Rate Label
   c. Pharmacy Label
III. Site Dressings and Changes
   a. Caring for the IV Site
   b. Changing the Dressing
IV. Complications and Risks
   a. Infiltration
   b. Extravasation
   c. Phlebitis
   d. Other Complications
V. Common Problems and Solutions
   a. IV Access
   b. Flow Rates
   c. IV Removal Problems

Learning Outcomes

- Identify the proper labeling technique for peripheral IV solutions, for medications given IVPB, and for blood products given intravenously.
- Apply, monitor, or replace an IV dressing when necessary.
- List the complications of IV therapy.
- Describe the signs and symptom of an infiltrated IV.
- Describe the signs and symptoms of a patient who has developed phlebitis from an IV.
- Describe the steps taken to prevent infiltration and phlebitis.
- List the common problems that can occur during IV therapy.
- Troubleshoot IV flow rate problems, including IVs that have stopped or are flowing too slow or too fast.
- Describe the steps taken to prevent bleeding or hematoma formation at an IV site.

Key Terms

blanching	hypersensitivity reaction
bronchospasm	infiltration
ecchymosis	phlebitis
erythema	sepsis
hematoma	vesicant

6-1 Introduction

Patients with IVs must have round-the-clock care. This constant care requires good communication with patients and with other staff members. When you start your shift, you need to be informed about what was done for a particular patient, just as the health care worker taking over from you needs to know what care you provided. Information that should be transmitted includes when the IV was started, whether it is infusing on schedule, and the condition of the IV site. The information that you obtain from the progress notes in the patient record and from the labels on the IV bag and the insertion site can help you determine when to change the infusion bag and tubing, when to redress or change the IV site, and whether the patient's IV site has developed complications such as infiltration or phlebitis.

Checkpoint Questions 6-1

1. What information do you need when you start to care for a patient with an IV?

_____

_____

2. Where do you find the information you need to care for a patient with an IV?

_____

_____

6-2 Labeling

Written communication in the form of accurate labels on the IV site, the tubing, and the solution bag facilitates patient care and reduces the chance for errors. Labels must be legible and must provide all relevant information about the cannula, dressing, solution, medication, and administration set. Proper labeling means that you do not have to leave the patient to check the medical record.

Site Label

As you learned in Chapter 5, when you start a new IV you must label the insertion site with the date and time the IV was started, the gauge and length of the catheter used, and your initials (Figure 6-1). By placing the insertion date on the IV site dressing label, you can easily determine when it is time to replace the IV catheter. Removing the catheter and restarting the IV in a

Figure 6-1 When an IV is started it must be labeled with the date, time, length and gauge of catheter, and initials. Frequently the label is written then placed on the patient's IV site.

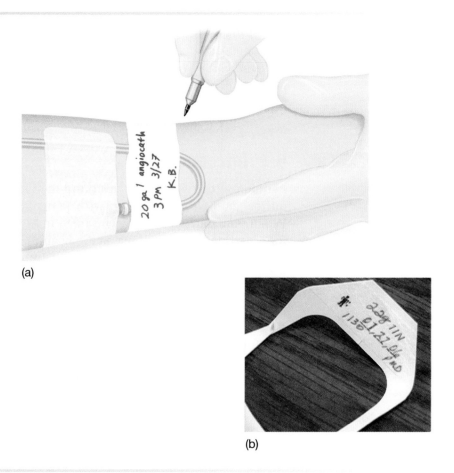

(a)

(b)

Figure 6-2 Tubing must be changed every 72 hours and should be labeled with the date, time, and initials of the person hanging the IV.

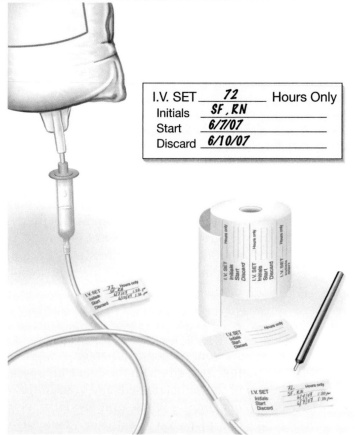

I.V. SET	*72*	Hours Only
Initials	*SF , RN*	
Start	*6/7/07*	
Discard	*6/10/07*	

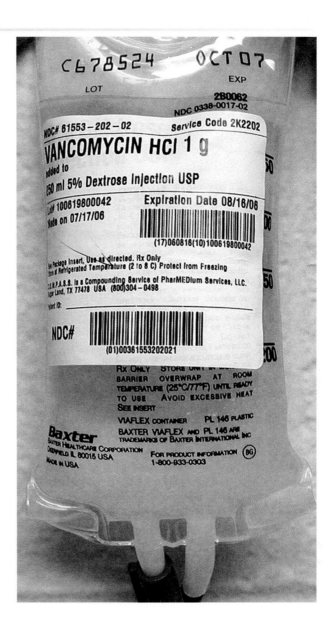

Figure 6-3 IV fluids are labeled by the manufacturer and by the pharmacy if medications are added.

different location should be done at least every 72 hours to reduce the incidence of infiltration or phlebitis. If you change the IV site dressing prior to restarting the IV, label the new dressing with all the original information plus the date of the dressing change.

Both the primary and the secondary IV sets must be labeled with the date and time they were hung and with your initials. You can do this quickly by placing a piece of tape around the tubing near the drip chamber (Figure 6-3).

Rate Label

All parenteral solutions are labeled with a rate label or a time-strip label that lists the name of the patient, the type of solution and any additives, the initials of the person hanging the bag, and the time the solution was started. Most IVs are administered with an infusion pump, but the time strip provides a quick reference for determining if the IV is infusing at the rate ordered. Commercial time strips have volume markings for a variety of IV

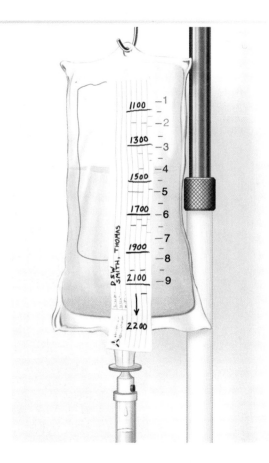

Figure 6-4 A time strip on the IV bag allows you to quickly determine if the infusion is flowing at the proper rate.

rates, and you simply write in the time at the appropriate volume marking (Figure 6-4). For example, if the IV is to infuse at 100 mL per hour and it is hung at 8:00 a.m., mark the time strip as starting at 8:00 a.m. with 1000 mL; at the 900 mL mark, write "9:00 a.m."; at the 800 mL mark, write "10:00 a.m."; and so forth. If a commercial rate label is not available, use a piece of tape with all required information.

Pharmacy Label

If the pharmacy prepares the IV solution, the bag will be labeled with the patient's name and unique identifier, the type and amount of solution, the type and amount of additive, the infusion rate, the date and time it is to be infused, the expiration date, and the initials of the pharmacist who prepared the admixture (Figure 6-2). IVs with this label still require a time strip that indicates the infusion rate.

IV infusions that contain medication are labeled with all the information listed in the previous paragraph plus the name and amount of medication. If you mix the medication for the IV solution bag, be sure that you label the bag properly and include your initials.

Secondary IV (piggyback) medication bags do not need a time strip because they are usually infused in less than an hour. If the medication is prepared in a bag greater than 100 mL and infuses longer than an hour, use a time strip to facilitate monitoring.

Check Fluids and Medications Three Times

Always check the IV fluid or medication label against the physician's order three times: (1) when it is obtained or taken off the shelf, (2) as you prepare it, and (3) prior to beginning the infusion.

Blood or blood products will come to your unit labeled for a specific patient. The bag itself will be labeled with the unit number, the type of blood product, the type of donor, the preservative, the expiration date, the blood type, and the Rh factor. An additional label or tag will have the patient's identifiers. Label the blood tubing and the IV site in the same manner that you would label all other IV infusions. When blood or blood products are administered, two licensed health care personnel must check the label before administration (Figure 6-5).

Figure 6-5   Blood Label.

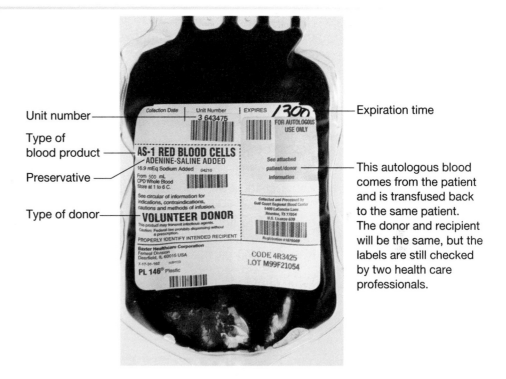

Unit number

Type of blood product

Preservative

Type of donor

Expiration time

This autologous blood comes from the patient and is transfused back to the same patient. The donor and recipient will be the same, but the labels are still checked by two health care professionals.

Checkpoint Questions 6-2

1. How do you properly label the IV site after changing a soiled dressing?

   _____

   _____

2. What is the purpose of the time strip on a peripheral IV solution?

   _____

   _____

Before you continue to the next section, answer the previous Checkpoint Questions and complete the Labeling activity under Chapter 6 on the student CD.

6-3 Site Dressings and Changes

Patients who receive IV therapy for more than 24 hours need to have their insertion site, tubing, fluid, and dressing changed at certain intervals to help prevent complications such as infection, infiltration, and phlebitis. The standards for IV therapy set by the Infusion Nurses Society (INS) are as follows:

- Peripheral IV sites are changed every 72 hours
- Tubing is changed every 72 hours with the site change
- A gauze dressing is changed every 48 hours; a transparent semipermeable membrane dressing is changed every 72 hours
- The solution is changed every 24 hours

If you ever encounter IV tubing or solution that is not labeled with a time and date and you cannot verify when the IV was hung, you should prepare and hang a new solution and tubing. By hanging a new IV, you reduce the possibility that the solution has infused longer than 24 hours and you avoid the complications that may arise, such as incompatibility.

Troubleshooting **Rising Cost VS Patient Care**

During the last staff meeting, your supervisor announced that because of rising costs, everyone must be careful about wasting medical supplies. Today when you checked a patient's IV, you observed that the bag and tubing were not labeled with the date and time they were hung. The IV is running at 50 mL/hour and still has 500 mL to infuse, so it will last through your shift.

What should you do?

_____

_____

Caring for the IV Site

The skin around the IV site is covered with a dressing made of sterile gauze and tape or of sterile transparent semipermeable membrane. Transparent semipermeable membrane dressings are used the most, because they provide the ability to see the IV site and also allow the patient to bathe. The standards require that membrane dressings be changed every 72 hours when the IV site is changed. Sterile gauze dressings are used when the patient is diaphoretic (sweaty) or when the site is oozing. According to standards, gauze dressings must be changed every 48 hours, which is more frequently than the site needs to be changed (Figure 6-6).

Each time you enter the patient's room, observe the patient's IV site. Look for moisture, oozing, or bleeding around or on the dressing. Check

Figure 6-6 (a) Gauze dressings are to be changed every 48 hours. (b) Semipermeable IV dressings are changed every 72 hours, usually at the same time the IV site is changed.

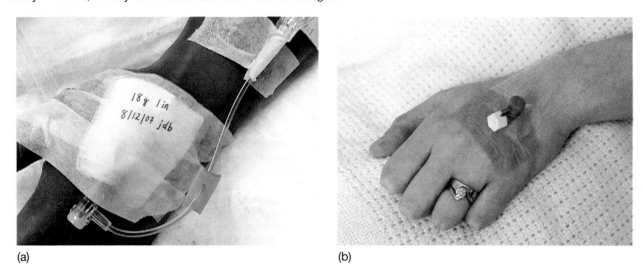

(a)   (b)

to make sure the dressing is not loose. Any loose, damp, or visibly soiled dressing should be changed immediately regardless of the recommended standards.

Changing the Dressing

The procedure for applying or changing an IV dressing varies, depending on the facility policy and on the type of equipment you are using. When applying a tape and sterile gauze dressing, place one piece of transparent tape under the catheter at the hub. Cross the tape over the hub and attach to the skin on the other side. Cross the other end of the tape in the opposite direction. Place a piece of sterile gauze under the hub of the needle and tape it in place. Avoid using nontransparent tape over the entry point of the catheter. The site should remain visible so you can check it for complications. Secure the IV in place with three or four strips of tape to prevent accidental removal. Place one or two pieces over the actual skin puncture site. Place additional pieces over loops of tubing to prevent any pulling or strain on the catheter when the patient moves. Consider taping to be one of your most important tasks because it prevents you from having to repeat the IV insertion in the event of an inadvertent tug on the IV tubing.

When applying a transparent semipermeable membrane dressing, check the directions on the dressing package first, because these products vary with the manufacturer. Peel off the backing from one side and smooth it across the site, removing additional backing while sealing the edges carefully. After attaching the membrane, make a small loop in the tubing near the insertion site and secure it over the dressing site. Tape the tubing as necessary depending on the location of the site and the possibility of accidental removal.

Regardless of whether you are applying a dressing for the first time or changing a dressing, always maintain the placement of the catheter. You must keep it stable while you are applying or removing any dressing, or your effort is lost. If the tubing is not connected, be certain to apply pressure over the vessel at the insertion site in order to prevent backflow of blood onto the dressing site.

1. What are the two types of dressings used for IV sites?

_____

_____

2. When should an IV dressing be changed?

_____

_____

Before you continue to the next section, answer the previous Checkpoint Questions and complete the Site Dressings and Changes activity under Chapter 6 on the student CD.

6-4 Complications and Risks

A number of complications can arise from IV therapy. Some are *localized*, meaning that they occur at or around the IV insertion site. Others are *systemic* complications that occur within the patient's vascular system, away from the insertion site. Systemic complications can be life-threatening.

TABLE 6-1 INS Infiltration Scale

Grade	Clinical Criteria
0	No symptoms
1	Skin blanched Edema < 1 in. around site Cool to touch With or without pain
2	Skin blanched Edema 1 to 6 in. around site Cool to touch With or without pain
3	Skin blanched and translucent Gross edema > 6 in. around site Cool to touch Mild to moderate pain Possible numbness
4	Skin blanched and translucent Skin tight, leaking Skin discolored, bruised, swollen Gross edema > 6 in. around site Deep pitting tissue edema Circulatory impairment Moderate to severe pain Infiltration of any amount of blood product, irritant, or vesicant

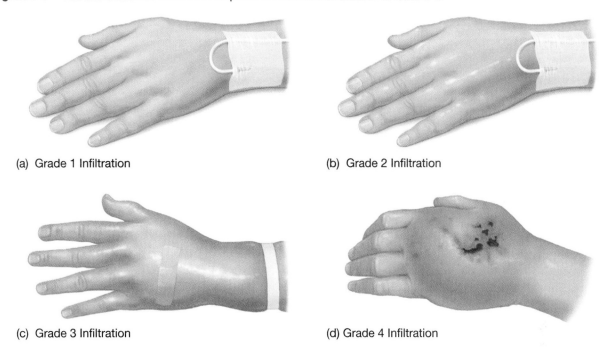

(a) Grade 1 Infiltration

(b) Grade 2 Infiltration

(c) Grade 3 Infiltration

(d) Grade 4 Infiltration

Infiltration

Infiltration is the inadvertent administration of a nonvesicant IV solution into surrounding tissue (Figure 6-7). A nonvesicant IV solution is one that does not cause blisters. Infiltration is a localized complication that occurs because the IV catheter is improperly placed or secured or becomes dislodged or because the veins are thin and fragile, as in elderly patients. The use of infusion pumps with a pressure setting greater than 10 psi (pounds per square inch) can also cause the IV to infiltrate. Signs and symptoms of infiltration include swelling, discomfort, burning, tightness, cool skin, and **blanching** (the whitish color that appears when pressure is applied to an area of the skin). The IV will not run, or it will run at a slower rate. If infiltration is severe, the patient can develop nerve and muscle damage and may lose function in the affected extremity.

Properly secure the IV to prevent dislodgment of the catheter or movement that may cause the catheter to puncture the vein wall. If the hand or arm with the IV is under the patient during patient turning, the IV may become occluded, causing the flow to back up and infiltrate. Careful monitoring of the IV insertion site can prevent infiltration. One way to determine if the IV has infiltrated is to apply slight pressure over the vein about three inches below the catheter tip; if the solution continues to run, it is probably infiltrated. Pressure over the vein below the catheter tip should occlude the vein and stop the infusing in an intact line (Figure 6-8).

Compare both arms of the patient for edema. If the arm with the IV appears larger, the IV may be infiltrated. However, immobilized or debilitated patients may have edema not related to the infiltration of an IV. You can check for a blood return, but it is not a reliable method of determining whether the IV is infiltrated, especially in veins that are fragile or have punctures from previous IVs or venipunctures.

Figure 6-8 To check if an IV is infiltrated, apply slight pressure over the vein about three inches below the catheter tip as marked in 6-8(a). If the IV stops infusing, it is intact and not infiltrated. For a gauze dressing you may need to estimate this location or remove the dressing.

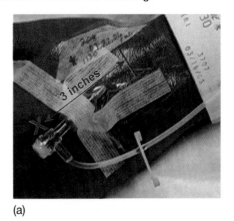

(a)

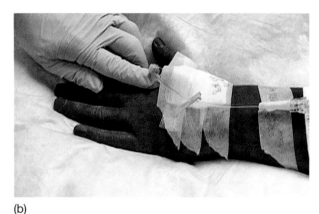

(b)

If infiltration occurs, stop the IV and remove the catheter. Determine the severity of infiltration by using the INS Infiltration Scale (see Table 6-1). A rating of Grade 2 or more should be reported as an unusual occurrence to the physician or your supervisor, and an incident report should be completed. Start a new IV in another site, usually the opposite arm. The severity of symptoms and the intervention depends on the amount and type of solution or medication that infiltrates into the tissues. If only a small amount of an isotonic solution or nonirritating medication infiltrates, patient discomfort is generally mild. Elevate the extremity slightly if patient desires, but elevation does not affect the rate of fluid reabsorption. Warm or cold compresses may be effective, depending on the solution that has infiltrated. Before applying warm or cold compresses, check your facility's policy to determine if a physician's order is required.

Extravasation

Extravasation occurs when **vesicant** drugs, such as some chemotherapeutic drugs, infiltrate a patient's IV insertion site (Figure 6-9). Extravasation can lead to severe tissue damage and requires emergency treatment. The causes of extravasation are the same as those for infiltration. The signs and symptoms are also the same, with the exception that vesicants will cause pain or burning around the IV site rather than just discomfort. Extravasation of a vesicant is

Figure 6-9 Infiltration from a vesicant fluid can cause extravasation, damaging the soft tissue in the area, as shown here.

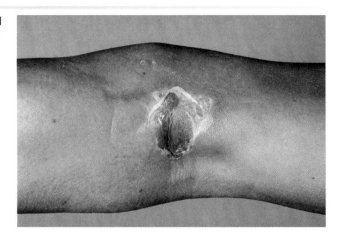

always rated as a Grade 4 on the INS Infiltration Scale regardless of the amount of fluid infiltrated. Stop the infusion immediately and replace the tubing, but do not remove the catheter because it may be needed to administer an antidote into the tissues. Remove the catheter only after the antidote is infused. Tissue damage from extravasation may produce an ulcer at the site and can lead to infection, disfigurement, loss of function, or amputation. Know your facility's established guidelines for the treatment of extravasation.

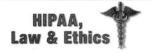

HIPAA, Law & Ethics

Monitor the IV Site

Monitor your patient's IV site carefully for complications. Long-term patient problems resulting from an IV complication such as phlebitis, infiltration, or extravasation can result in lawsuits for medical negligence or malpractice.

Phlebitis

Phlebitis is an inflammation of the vein due to mechanical or chemical causes (Figure 6-10). Mechanical causes include using a large catheter in a small vein, improperly securing the catheter and thereby allowing movement, and overmanipulating the IV catheter. Prolonged use of the same IV site increases the patient's risk of developing phlebitis. Chemical phlebitis is caused by irritating or vesicant medications or by solutions that are acidic or alkaline or that have a high osmolarity. Some common medications and solutions that are irritating are

- Erythromycin
- Nafcillin sodium
- Vancomycin
- Amphotericin B
- Potassium chloride

Chemical phlebitis can also be caused by particulates in the solution, such as medications that do not fully dissolve but are not visible to the eye. Using a filter can eliminate this factor. Sometimes the catheter itself can cause phlebitis. Silicone and polyurethane catheters are smoother and less irritating than those made of Teflon. Intermittent infusions of heparin or saline lock devices are less irritating to the vein than continuous infusions are. If the patient can tolerate the extra fluid, it may be useful to add extra diluent to the infusion. Slowing the infusion rate of irritating solutions may also reduce the possibility of phlebitis. Start IVs in larger veins using the smallest catheter appropriate for the solution. Because phlebitis may occur after two to three days of continuous IV therapy, replace peripheral catheters every 72 hours. Use central lines for long-term IV therapies. Be aware that phlebitis can develop 48 to 96 hours after removal of an IV cannula without the usual signs and symptoms, so check previous IV sites for several days after cannula removal.

Signs and symptoms of phlebitis include **erythema** (redness) and/or tenderness at the tip of the device, puffiness over the vein, skin that is warm to the touch at the IV site, a slowed infusion rate, and an elevated temperature. INS recommends using the Phlebitis Scale to evaluate the site

Figure 6-10 The INS classifies phlebitis as pictured here and described in table 6-2.

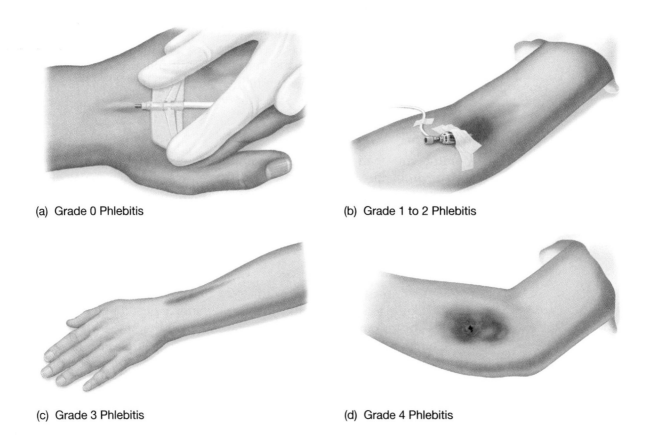

(a) Grade 0 Phlebitis

(b) Grade 1 to 2 Phlebitis

(c) Grade 3 Phlebitis

(d) Grade 4 Phlebitis

(see Table 6-2). As with infiltration, a phlebitis rating of Grade 2 or higher should be reported as an unusual occurrence to the physician or your supervisor, and an incident report should be completed. If phlebitis at Grade 1 or higher occurs, stop the infusion and remove the device. Apply warm or cold compresses after checking your facility's policy to determine if a

TABLE 6-2 **INS Phlebitis Scale**

Grade	Clinical Criteria
0	No symptoms
1	Erythema at access site with or without pain
2	Pain at access site with erythema and/or edema
3	Pain at access site with erythema and/or edema Streak formation Palpable venous cord
4	Pain at access site with erythema and/or edema Streak formation Palpable venous cord Purulent drainage

physician's order is required. Be sure to notify the physician about phlebitis with a rating of Grade 3 or 4. If caught early, phlebitis can be easily treated, so it is important to check the site frequently. If not caught early, phlebitis can cause local infection, severe discomfort, and possibly **sepsis.** Sepsis is a serious systemic infection that is life-threatening.

Patient Education & Communication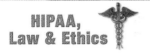

Report Complications Immediately

Instruct your patients to immediately report any discomfort, swelling, or redness at an IV site.

HIPAA, Law & Ethics

Incidence Report

An incident report must be completed if an occurrence of infiltration or phlebitis is rated Grade 2 or higher on the appropriate INS scale. An incident report must be completed on all cases of extravasation. Incident reports document the problem and how it was treated, and also provide information for preventing the problem in the future.

Other Complications

Although infiltration and phlebitis are the more common complications of IV therapy, there are several other problems that you must watch for. Patients on IV therapy may develop a fluid overload. Fluid overload occurs because the patient has received too much solution or is not able to tolerate increased amounts of fluid. Symptoms include respiratory distress (difficulty breathing), neck vein distension, and increased blood pressure. If a patient becomes overloaded, slow the infusion to a keep-open rate and notify the physician. You may want to place the patient in a semi-Fowler's position to ease the respiratory distress. In the semi-Fowler's position, the patient is on his or her back and the head of the bed or table is elevated at least 45 degrees. The physician will order diuretics to remove the excess fluid and oxygen to improve respiratory status.

Always watch for the possibility that the patient will have a **hypersensitivity reaction** (allergic reaction) even if the patient reported no known allergies. To decrease the chance of a hypersensitivity reaction, check both with the patient and the patient's medical record for information about allergies or a family history of allergies. Observe the patient closely, especially during administration of the first dose of any new medication. Signs and symptoms of a hypersensitivity reaction include

- Rash, itching
- Tearing eyes, runny nose
- **Bronchospasm** (constriction of the air passages)
- Wheezing
- Anaphylaxis

If the patient exhibits any unusual symptoms during the infusion, stop the medication immediately and notify the physician. Maintain the vascular access device, either with the continuous IV or as a saline lock. Make sure the patient has an open airway and support respirations if reaction is severe. Epinephrine, antihistamines, and steroids are the typical treatment for a hypersensitivity reaction.

Patients receiving IV therapy must be closely monitored for infection. Untreated, a local infection at an IV site can lead to systemic infection or sepsis because pathogens have direct access to the blood. If the site is extremely red and has any purulent drainage, it is probably infected. Stop the IV infusion, remove the catheter, and notify the physician. A culture of the drainage should be ordered, and if policy dictates, the catheter can also be cultured. Watch the patient closely for the possibility of sepsis. Antibiotics may be ordered.

Safety and Infection Control

Always Follow Standard Precautions

The patient's risk of developing an infection at an IV site can be reduced if you follow the Standard Precautions guidelines when starting an IV and performing routine site care.

Patients with an IV, especially a central line IV, may develop an air embolus, which is when air enters the heart and causes it to work harder. Air may enter the IV system when the catheter and tubing become separated. Untreated, an air embolus can lead to decreased cardiac output, shock, and death. Symptoms include respiratory distress and possible mid-chest and shoulder pain. The patient may also complain of nausea and lightheadedness. An air embolus is an emergency situation. Close off the catheter immediately by using the slide clamp or by folding the tubing over on itself. Place the patient on the left side, head down. This position keeps the air bubble in the right atrium and prevents it from moving into the pulmonary artery. Start the patient on oxygen and notify the physician because prompt medical care is necessary.

Checkpoint Questions 6-4

1. What are the possible complications of IV therapy?

   _____

   _____

2. What is the difference between infiltration and phlebitis?

   _____

   _____

 Before you continue to the next section, answer the previous Checkpoint Questions and complete the Complications and Risks activity under Chapter 6 on the student CD.

6-5 Common Problems and Solutions

Problems with IV therapy can occur throughout the process, from insertion to removal. Three common problems that you will encounter are (1) the IV is difficult to insert, (2) the IV may not infuse at the correct rate, and (3) the IV site may develop problems after the IV is removed. The rest of this section offers solutions to these common problems.

Whenever you encounter complications with an IV, you must take corrective action immediately to decrease further risks and to prevent prolonging the infusion. Document the problem encountered, the actions taken, and the patient response. For example, you might write, "IV alarm sounding frequently. IV flow rate appears to slow with movement of the wrist. Small wrist board applied. Patient instructed to keep wrist straight as possible during infusion."

IV Access

Not all patients have easily accessible veins. Conditions that may lead to difficult venous access include skin lesions or rashes, sclerosing (hard) veins, obesity, and edema. In addition, elderly patients frequently have fragile veins that make access and continued therapy difficult. Direct a light toward the side of the extremity to improve the visibility of veins in patients with alterations in the skin (rashes, dermatitis) or with dark skin (Figure 6-11).

Patients with sclerosing veins present a special problem. Use a smaller vein if the patient has good circulation. Otherwise, this patient may require a central line if no adequate peripheral lines are available. The veins of obese patients may either be shallow because they have been displaced by the adipose tissue, or they may be buried deep in the tissue. Shallow veins present no special problem, but to access deep veins, you must use a longer catheter (at least 2 in.). You learned in Chapter 5 how to locate a suitable vein in a patient with edema. Displace the tissue fluid by pressing on the access site. Insert the catheter quickly to prevent the fluid from returning and making the site difficult to see. After you insert the catheter, you must also be sure that pressure from the edema in the tissues does not cause the vein to collapse, stopping the infusion. You may have to move the IV to a less edematous site or to a larger vein, such as the antecubital vein. For elderly patients or any patient with fragile veins, use the smallest gauge catheter possible and lower the angle of insertion. Stabilize the vein by pulling the skin tight. To prevent overdistending and rupturing fragile veins, do not apply the tourniquet more than 1 to 2 minutes before you are ready to start the IV, and do not apply the tourniquet too tightly.

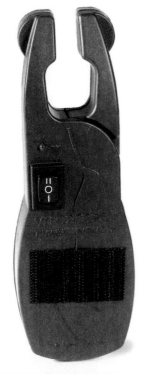

Figure 6-11 A special light can be used to improve the visibility of veins in patients with rashes, dermatitis, or dark skin.

Flow Rates

The most common problems with IV infusions are related to infusion (flow) rates. Poorly regulated infusions can lead to fluid overload, overdosing or underdosing of a medication, clogged IV catheters, phlebitis, and infiltration. Factors that play a role in flow rate control may be patient-related, equipment-related, or vein-related.

One patient-related factor is the patient's blood pressure. A slower infusion rate—such as a KVO infusion of 10mL/hr—may be difficult to maintain in a patient with high blood pressure. A gravity drip may not be able to overcome the high pressure in the vascular system, so use an infusion pump to maintain the correct rate. Sometimes the patient or family members make adjustments in the IV rate. You may be able to eliminate this problem through patient and family education. If not, use an infusion pump with a locking mechanism to prevent the patient or family members from altering the flow rate.

Equipment-related problems such as clogged filters or kinked IV tubing can slow or stop the infusion. A solution with a higher viscosity or thickness may run slower. The roller clamp may slip, resulting in a faster rate. Even the height of the IV pole can affect the flow rate. If the IV pole is raised after the initial drip rate is set, the flow rate will increase. Lowering the IV pole will slow the rate. (If an infusion pump is used, however, pole adjustments will have no effect on flow rate.) Warm solutions drip faster than cold solutions do. Refrigerated solutions should be warmed to room temperature prior to hanging. If you set the flow rate while the solution is cold, you will have to reset the rate once the solution warms to room temperature. The flow rate may be slowed because the catheter is against the vein wall or the patient's arm may be bent. All these problems have simple solutions (see Table 6-3). Troubleshoot the cause of changes in flow rate and make adjustments accordingly. If the flow is too fast, adjust the regulator to the correct drip rate and continue the infusion. Observe the patient for signs of fluid overload or medication overdosing. If the flow is too slow, the patient is not receiving the correct amount of medication or solution, and the IV catheter can clog, requiring a restart. If the flow is too slow, *do not* speed up the IV flow rate in order to "catch up." If rate has been too slow or too fast, recalculate the flow rate based on the amount of solution remaining and the time remaining from the original order.

Most problems with infusion pumps are due to air in the line, to kinked or obstructed tubing, or to occluded catheters. When an infusion pump's alarm sounds, follow the manufacturer's troubleshooting guide. These guides are either attached to or directly on the pumps for easy reference.

Patient Education & Communication

Infusion Pumps

Instruct your patient and the patient's family members about the function and use of the infusion pump and what they should do when an alarm sounds. Explain that the pump should not be turned off or the settings changed by anyone without proper instruction. The result could be the loss of the IV site or the administration of an incorrect amount of fluid or medication.

Vein-related problems include infiltration, phlebitis, and venous spasm. Infiltration and phlebitis cause the flow rate to decrease. See discussions earlier in this chapter for prevention and treatment of these complications. Venous spasm is the contraction of a vein that causes the blood to stop flowing through the vessel. It can result from the infusion of cold or irritating solutions or from a solution that infuses too fast. If a spasm occurs, the flow rate will slow or stop and the patient will complain of a sharp pain that starts at the IV site and moves up the extremity. You can prevent venous spasm if you dilute additives properly, warm refrigerated solutions before infusing, and maintain proper flow rates.

TABLE 6-3 Troubleshooting Flow Rate Problems

Problem	Solution
Flow rate in primary line is too slow.	• Check the roller (flow rate) clamp; reset it by counting the drip rate or drops per minute (gtt/min) of the IV flow • Check for kinks or bends in the tubing • Check the height of the IV bag • Reposition the catheter because it may be up against the vein wall • Reposition the patient's extremity • Check for signs of phlebitis or infiltration • Change the filter if there is one • Recalculate and reset the infusion rate
Flow rate in primary line is too fast.	• Check the roller (flow rate) clamp; reset it by counting the drip rate or drops per minute (gtt/min) of the IV flow • Check the height of the IV bag • Recalculate and reset the infusion rate • Place on an infusion pump if strict control is needed
IV flow in primary line has stopped.	• Check the roller (flow rate) clamp; reset it by counting the drip rate or the drops per minute (gtt/min) of the IV flow • Check for signs of phlebitis or infiltration • Check for blood return • Change the filter if there is one • Use a thrombolytic to unclot the catheter (if facility policy permits)
Flow rate in secondary set is too slow or has stopped.	• Check that the primary bag is lower than the secondary bag • Check the solutions in the primary IV line

Infusion pump alarm sounds and a message is displayed:
  Infusion complete
  Occlusion
  Low battery
  Cassette
  Air in line
	Follow the manufacturer's instructions for troubleshooting alarms.
	
	• Hang a new IV solution bag; the volume limit has been reached
	• Check the insertion site; check for kinks in tubing; check for closed clamps
	• Plug the machine into an outlet
	• Reload the medication cassette
	• Flush the line to clear out the air

IV Removal Problems

Bleeding and hematoma can occur when an IV catheter is removed. You may encounter these problems if you do not hold pressure on the site long enough after removing the catheter. Holding the site is especially important for patients who are taking anticoagulants. Bleeding from discontinued IV sites can be small amounts that ooze or larger amounts that flow from the site. A **hematoma** is a mass of partially clotted blood that has infiltrated into the tissues; it is usually accompanied by **ecchymosis,** a bruising of the skin surrounding the puncture site. Symptoms include swelling and discomfort at the site. Prevent both bleeding and hematomas by applying direct pressure over the IV site for 2 to 3 minutes with a sterile gauze pad after the catheter is removed. You may elevate the arm over the patient's head or on a pillow. If a hematoma develops, apply ice packs to prevent its enlargement, but check your facility's policy because a physician's order may be needed. A site with a hematoma and ecchymosis cannot be used again until the hematoma and bruising have resolved.

Checkpoint Questions 6-5

1. If you observe that an IV is running too slow or too fast, what actions should you take?

_____

_____

2. List the three factors that can cause rate problems related to IV infusions.

_____

_____

 Before you continue to the chapter summary, answer the previous Checkpoint Questions and complete the Common Problems and Solutions activity under Chapter 6 on the student CD.

Chapter Summary

- IV setups are labeled in three places: by the insertion site, on the tubing, and on the solution bag. Labels include the date and time of the infusion; information relative to the cannula, solution, or additives; and the initials of the health care provider who performs the care.

- IV dressings are made of sterile gauze and tape or a semipermeable transparent membrane. Dressings are changed on schedule or when soiled or loose.

- Complications of IV therapy include infiltration, phlebitis, extravasation, fluid overload, hypersensitivity reaction, infection, air embolus, insertion difficulties, and bleeding or hematoma on removal of the catheter.

- Signs and symptoms of an infiltrated IV include swelling, discomfort, burning, tightness, cool skin, and blanching.

- Signs and symptoms of phlebitis include erythema (redness) and/or tenderness at the tip of the device, puffiness over the vein, warmth, a slowed flow rate, and an elevated temperature.

- Infiltration and phlebitis can be prevented if the IV is closely monitored and properly secured. The proper-sized catheter should be used, and manipulation of the site should be minimized.

- Common problems in IV therapy occur because of poor veins, unregulated flow rates, and improper discontinuation of an IV.

- Erratic flow rates are the most common problem of IV therapy. Poorly regulated infusions can lead to fluid overload, overdosing or underdosing of medications, clogged IV catheters, infiltration, and phlebitis. Factors in flow rate alterations may be patient-related, equipment-related, or vein-related. The cause must be corrected and the correct flow rate reestablished.

- Bleeding or hematoma at an IV site can be prevented if direct pressure is applied to the site for 2 to 3 minutes when the catheter is removed; arm elevation can also help.

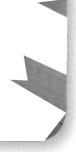

Matching

_____ **1.** erythema

_____ **2.** hypersensitivity reaction

_____ **3.** infiltration

_____ **4.** vesicant

_____ **5.** phlebitis

_____ **6.** extravasation

a. inflammation of the inner lining of a vein associated with chemical or mechanical irritation or bacterial infection

b. a medication or agent that produces blisters

c. redness of the skin resulting from inflammation

d. leakage of a vesicant fluid from a vessel into the surrounding tissue

e. seepage of IV fluids into surrounding tissues

f. allergic reaction; response of the immune system to a medication, solution, or other substance

True/False

T   F   **7.** IV labels must be legible and must provide all relevant information.

T   F   **8.** Phlebitis is the leakage of vesicant fluids into tissues surrounding an IV site.

T   F   **9.** The correct way to determine if an IV has infiltrated is to check for a blood return in the tubing.

T   F   **10.** Blood pressure can affect the flow rate of an IV.

T   F   **11.** Direct pressure applied to an IV site after the removal of the catheter can prevent bleeding or hematoma.

Multiple Choice

12. What information should you put on the tubing label?
   a. insertion date and time, size of the catheter, initials
   b. date and time hung, initials
   c. additives, date and time hung, initials
   d. insertion date and time, additives, initials

13. What is the purpose of the time strip placed on IV solution bags?
   a. to identify the patient
   b. to regulate the IV
   c. to help determine if the IV is on schedule
   d. to prevent a medication error

14. What information is required on a label for an IVPB medication?
    a. patient name, name and amount of solution
    b. name and amount of medication
    c. infusion time, initials of preparer
    d. all of the above

15. Which of the following factors increases the possibility of complications from IV therapy?
    a. solutions that hang more than 12 hours and catheters that are in place less than 48 hours
    b. solutions that hang less than 24 hours and catheters that are changed every 48 hours
    c. solutions that hang longer than 24 hours and catheters that are in place longer than 72 hours
    d. solutions that hang longer than 24 hours and catheters that are in place less than 72 hours

16. Which of the following are the signs and symptoms of an infiltrated IV?
    a. swelling, discomfort, tightness, cool skin, blanching, slow or stopped flow rate
    b. swelling, redness, tightness, cool skin, blanching, slow or stopped flow rate
    c. bruising, discomfort, tightness, cool skin, blanching, slow or stopped flow rate
    d. severe pain, swelling, tightness, cool skin, blanching, slow or stopped flow rate

17. Which of these agents can cause extravasation?
    a. erythromycin
    b. normal saline
    c. vesicants
    d. heparin

18. Which of the following can cause phlebitis?
    a. prolonged use of the same catheter site, use of irritating solutions
    b. use of a catheter too large for the vein
    c. both a and b
    d. neither a nor b

19. Which of the following are the patient-related factors that play a role in flow rate control?
    a. sepsis and high blood pressure
    b. blood pressure and rate changes made by a family member
    c. height of the IV pole and temperature of the solution
    d. position of the IV and viscosity of the solution

20. Which of the following may cause an IV to run too slow?
    a. IV pole was raised after the drip rate was set
    b. regulator is set too high
    c. tubing is kinked under the patient
    d. none of the above

21. Which of the following medications increases the chance of bleeding when an IV is removed?
    a. insulin
    b. ampicillin
    c. potassium
    d. heparin

What Should You Do? (Critical Thinking/Application Questions)

1. Your patient is complaining of pain at his IV site. When you inspect the site, you find that the transparent dressing is intact and the site is red but not swollen. You note that the flow rate is correct, and you notice no red streaks at the site. What should you do? How would you chart your action?

_____

_____

_____

2. Your patient's IV is being administered with an infusion pump. The pump's alarm is sounding intermittently, and the pump displays the message "line occluded." What actions would you take to correct the problem?

_____

_____

_____

Get Connected

Visit the McGraw-Hill Higher Education website for _Intravenous Therapy for Health Care Personnel_ at **www.mhhe.com/healthcareskills** to complete the following activities.

1. Take a trip to the IV Team website from the link provided on the website for _Intravenous Therapy for Health Care Personnel_. Click on IV Pictures and view the various complications of IV therapy. Select three complications and write a brief summary of how they can be prevented.

 ## Using the Student CD

Now that you have completed the material in Chapter 6, return to the student CD and complete any chapter activities you have not yet done. Practice your terminology with the Key Term Concentration game. Review the chapter material with the Spin the Wheel game. Take the final chapter test, complete the troubleshooting question, and e-mail or print your results to document your proficiency for this chapter.

7 Documenting and Discontinuation

Chapter Outline

I. Introduction
II. Documenting IV Therapy
  a. Documentation after IV Initiation
  b. Documentation during IV Therapy
  c. Documentation after IV Discontinuation
  d. Abbreviations in Documentation
III. Monitoring IV Therapy
IV. Documenting Fluid Balance
  a. Intake and Output
  b. Documenting Fluids
V. Discontinuing an IV

Learning Outcomes

- Identify when documentation of intravenous therapy must be done.
- Describe proper documentation for IV initiation, during IV therapy, and for IV discontinuation.
- State the importance of avoiding ambiguous abbreviations or terms in documentation.
- Identify information that must be documented and/or reported when monitoring IV therapy.
- List what must be documented for intake and output during IV therapy.
- Differentiate between the terms *IV to be absorbed (TBA)* and *IV absorbed*.
- Discuss the procedure for discontinuing a peripheral IV infusion.

Key Terms

anticoagulants
intake and output (I&O)
intake and output (I&O) record
IV absorbed
IV to be absorbed (TBA)
urometer

152

7-1 Introduction

Documentation is necessary for all patient care. If information about the care is not recorded, the care is not considered done. Both lack of documentation and inaccurate documentation can cause problems for health care employees. The facility at which you are employed, health care regulating agencies, and lawyers handling malpractice lawsuits all expect you to have properly documented any procedure that you perform.

Discontinuation of IV therapy is done with the aseptic technique and must be documented completely. You must correctly perform the discontinuation procedure in order to prevent pain and complications in the patient. In some situations, it may be within your scope of practice to discontinue an IV even if you are not permitted to initiate an IV. As always, perform only those procedures that are within your scope of practice.

Checkpoint Question 7-1

1. Why must complete and accurate documentation be done for all patient care and procedures?

_____

_____

7-2 Documenting IV Therapy

Every health care facility requires accurate and complete documentation of IV infusion. Standards for intravenous therapy are set by JCAHO, and guidelines for documentation are established by each health care facility. Documentation forms and frequency requirements will vary, but the information that is documented is generally the same. Documentation of IV therapy is required after the initiation of venous access, during the course of treatment, and when the IV is discontinued (Figure 7-1).

Documentation after IV Initiation

As you learned in Chapter 5, when you insert an IV, you must document the size and type of catheter, the number of attempts, the date and time, the site of insertion, the type of solution and additives or medications, the flow rate, the pump information (if appropriate), the type of dressing applied, and your name or initials. You must also label the solution, the tubing, and the dressing. Remember, only the person who starts the IV should chart this information.

Some facilities allow you to document your number of attempts by simply placing a mark on an anatomical drawing of the extremity. You may also document the insertion by naming the vein or the location and providing a thorough description of the exact placement along the vein and extremity.

Include in your documentation any patient education that you provided. Some facilities provide flow charts that have a patient education section. If you have such a chart, use it to describe the patient education you provided; otherwise, chart the information in the narrative notes. For example chart "Pt instructed on reason for IV, signs and symptoms to report, activity level, and pump alarms."

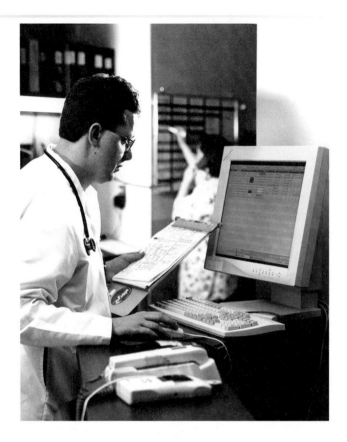

Figure 7-1 Each facility sets standards for documentation. In many facilities, all documentation is done electronically.

Documentation during IV Therapy

During IV therapy, always document any site care that you give, such as changing the IV dressing. Include the condition and appearance of the site as well as the patient's response. Whenever you replace a fluid container, document the condition of the site and the condition of the patient.

Your facility may require hourly, daily, and/or shift assessments that include information about the IV infusion as well as any unusual signs and symptoms. See Table 7-1 for a list of recommended items to document when you are monitoring and maintaining an IV infusion.

Documentation after IV Discontinuation

When you discontinue an IV, look closely at the insertion site and document what you observe. Include information about the patient's response to the procedure; if possible, use an exact quote of the patient's comments. Record the following information in the patient's medical record:

- the date and time the IV was discontinued,
- the reason for discontinuation,
- the condition of the catheter,
- and whether the catheter was intact (complete).

This last piece of information is very important because a portion of a catheter that has been sheared off and left in the vein can cause a catheter embolus, which is potentially fatal. *If the catheter is not intact, place a tourniquet above the infusion site and notify the physician immediately.*

Be sure to document whether you used an arm board, and state why the board was used. *This documentation should also have been done when*

TABLE 7-1   Documentation Recommendations

Component	Items to Be Documented
Fluid	Volume and composition
Intake and output	Intake: IV, oral, tube feeding Output: urine, diarrhea, drainage
Signs and symptoms of fluid overload	• Eyes: orbital edema • Skin: warm to the touch; moist-dependent edema • Respiratory system: dyspnea; crackles; wheezing; increased respiration rate; pulmonary edema • Cardiac system: bounding pulse; vein distension
Signs and symptoms of fluid deficit	• Eyes: dry conjunctiva; reduced tearing; sunken appearance • Mouth: dry, sticky mucous membranes; dry, cracked lips • Skin: diminished turgor • Neurologic system: reduced central nervous system activity • Cardiac system: narrowed pulse pressure; lowered blood pressure • Weight loss • Fever; source and amount of any body fluid loss
Electrolyte imbalance	• Sodium excess: lowered urine output (oliguria); increased body temperature • Sodium deficit: increased viscosity of saliva; increased urine volume; all mental status changes; signs and symptoms of increased intracranial pressure, such as headache and increased blood pressure • Potassium excess: irregular heart rate; diminished urine volume; ECG changes • Potassium deficit: muscle weakness; cardiac arrhythmias

the arm board was placed on the patient. Follow-up measures, such as application of a dressing or the restart of an IV at another site, should also be documented.

Look for any signs of inflammation or infection at the catheter site, and note whether the patient exhibits symptoms of infection. *If you see any indication of infection, you must take necessary and appropriate action to protect the patient.* Because IV therapy is invasive and can lead to infection, any sign of infection usually requires that the catheter tip be cultured to identify any bacteria. To prepare a catheter for culture when you discontinue an IV, cut off the tip of the catheter with sterile scissors and place it in a sterile container before you dispose of the IV administration set. Prepare a lab slip or lab requisition requesting the culture, and send the container to the lab (Figure 7-2). Document this procedure in the patient's medical record as "catheter tip sent to the lab."

Abbreviations in Documentation

When documenting IV therapy, avoid using dangerous or ambiguous abbreviations because these can lead to medication errors. For example, never use

Figure 7-2 Laboratory requisition for the culture of an IV catheter tip.

LABORATORY REQUISITION

| FOR CLIENT USE ONLY: Requisition Date:_____ | FOR PATH USE ONLY: | Path #_____ |
| Completed By: _____ Accn# _____ | Record _____ | |

PART A - PATIENT INFORMATION - *Required*
Patient Name:
Street:
City: St: Zip:
Phone: (   )
Date of Birth: Gender: Male   Female
Social Security #:

PART B - PROVIDER INFORMATION - *Required*
Referring Institution:
Street:
City: St: Zip:
Phone: Fax:
Referring Physician:
Referring Physician UPIN:

PART C) SPECIMEN INFORMATION

Date Collected: _07_ / _11_ / _07_   Time: _1421_

Specimen Type: ☐ Serum ☐ Plasma ☐ Whole Blood
☐ Random Urine   24 hr. Urine – volume:_____
☒ Other (specify): _IV CATHETER TIP_

TEST(S) REQUESTED: (Please include or attach any additional information such as specimen specifics or pertinent clinical history)

CULTURE CATHETER TIP FROM DISCONTINUED IV
— IV SITE RED, WARM, EDEMATOUS

**REFER TO OUR TEST DIRECTORY HANDBOOK FOR SPECIMEN REQUIREMENTS
AND HANDLING INSTRUCTIONS**

PART D - SEND BILL TO:

Referring Institution (Applies to ALL In-Patient Consultations)
Patient's Insurance (Complete billing information must be provided or referring institution may be billed)

Primary Insurance Coverage Information	Secondary Insurance Coverage Information
Insured by: _____	Insured by: _____
Claims Address: _____	Claims Address: _____
City : _____ ST:_____ Zip: _____	City : _____ ST:_____ Zip: _____
Policy/ID #: _____ Group #: _____	Policy/ID #: _____ Group #: _____
Name of Subscriber: _____	Name of Subscriber: _____
Relationship to Patient: _____	Relationship to Patient: _____
Required ICD-9 codes: 1. ____ 2. ____ 3. ____	4. ____ 5. ____

Authorization/Referral #_____

If the guarantor is someone other than the patient, guarantor
information is required. Please supply the guarantor information to
the right. ————————————▶

Guarantor Name:
Guarantor Address:

Medicare will only pay for the services that it determines to be "reasonable and necessary" under section 1862(a)(1) of the Medicare Law. If Medicare determines that a particular service, although it would otherwise be covered, is not "reasonable and necessary" under the Medicare standards, Medicare will deny payment for that service or test.

the letter "U" as an abbreviation for "unit." It can easily be misread as the number four or as a zero, which would make the dose appear to be 10 times greater than intended. Always write out the word "units." JCAHO has developed a complete list of abbreviations that should be avoided and has placed on each health care organization the responsibility for devising a plan to institute and monitor compliance with abbreviation use. JCAHO's do-not-use abbreviations and undesirable abbreviations are listed in Tables 7-2 and 7-3. When you are documenting IV therapy, use only the abbreviations recognized by your facility and approved by JCAHO.

TABLE 7-2 Do-Not-Use Abbreviations

Abbreviation	Potential Problem	Preferred Term
U (for unit)	Mistaken as a zero, a four, or "cc"	Write "unit"
IU (for international unit)	Mistaken as "IV" (intravenous) or "10" (ten)	Write "international unit"
Q.D. Q.O.D. (Latin abbreviations for "once daily" and "every other day")	Mistaken for each other; the period after the Q can be mistaken for an "I"; the "O" can be mistaken for an "I"	Write "daily" and "every other day"
Trailing zero* ("X.0 mg") Lack of leading zero (".X mg")	Decimal point is missed	Never write a zero by itself after a decimal point ("X mg"); always use a zero before a decimal point ("0.X mg")
MS MSO_4 $MgSO_4$	Mistaken for one another; can mean "morphine sulfate" or "magnesium sulfate"	Write "morphine sulfate" or "magnesium sulfate"

*Prohibited only for medication-related notations.

TABLE 7-3 Undesirable Abbreviations

Abbreviation	Potential Problem	Preferred Term
μg (symbol for "microgram")	Mistaken as "mg" (milligrams), resulting in a one-thousand-fold overdose	Write "mcg"
H.S. (for "half-strength" or Latin abbreviation for "bedtime")	Mistaken for each other; "q.H.S." mistaken for "every hour"; all can result in a dosing error	Write "half-strength" or "at bedtime"
T.I.W. (for "three times a week")	Mistaken as "three times a day" or "twice weekly," resulting in an overdose	Write "3 times weekly" or "three times weekly"
S.C. S.Q. (for "subcutaneous")	Mistaken as "S.L." (sublingual) or "five every"	Write "sub-Q" or "subQ" or "subcutaneously"
D/C (for "discharge")	Interpreted as "discontinue [whatever medications follow, typically discharge meds]"	Write "discharge"
cc (for "cubic centimeter")	Mistaken as "U" (units)	Write "mL" (for "milliliters")
A.S. A.D. A.U. (Latin abbreviations for "left ear," "right ear," "both ears")	Mistaken as "O.S." (left eye), "O.D." (right eye), "O.U." (both eyes)	Write "left ear," "right ear," "both ears"

1. When should IV therapy be documented?

_____

_____

2. You have just completed your assessment on a patient who has IV fluids infusing. What items must be included in your documentation?

_____

_____

Before you continue to the next section, answer the previous Checkpoint Questions and complete the Documenting IV Therapy activity under Chapter 7 on the student CD.

7-3 Monitoring IV Therapy

Successfully initiating an IV is only the beginning of your responsibility in providing proper IV therapy for your patients. You must monitor your well-placed cannula regularly so that your patients can meet the objectives of their treatment plans. Being an observant care provider will help you intervene early to prevent harm to your patients. Document your observations, and report problems to the physician or your supervisor so appropriate action can be taken.

Recall from Chapter 6 that pain or swelling near the IV insertion site may indicate infiltration or phlebitis. Infiltration is also indicated by swelling, discomfort, and coolness at the site as well as a sizable decrease in flow rate. Pain at the IV site is the most common sign of phlebitis. Other signs include heat, redness, and swelling at the insertion site. Regularly take the patient's vital signs, and watch for hypertension or shortness of breath. If you encounter any problems, you must document them and take necessary action. See Table 7-4 for more information.

Troubleshooting

Handling a Problem with an IV

The patient just had his IV started a few hours ago and is complaining that the IV site is hurting. You check the IV and notice that it is running on schedule and has no redness or swelling. What would be your best course of action at this point in the patient care?

_____

_____

TABLE 7-4 Documenting IV Problems

Problem	Documentation	Possible Cause	Action
Site is red, sore, swollen; patient is febrile	Document the patient's actual temperature; document the patient's amount of pain ranked on a pain scale of 1 to 10	Infection	Notify supervisor
Site is swollen, cool to the touch, taut, uncomfortable for patient; IV has stopped or is sluggish	Document the patient's amount of pain ranked on a pain scale of 1 to 10; document the rate of flow	Infiltration	Notify supervisor
Site is sore, hard, warm; red line appears above site; IV is sluggish or has stopped	Document the patient's amount of pain ranked on a pain scale of 1 to 10; document the rate of flow	Clot formation	Notify supervisor immediately
IV has infused ahead of schedule; patient is short of breath, has increased respirations, has increased blood pressure	Document patient's respiratory rate and blood pressure; document the patient's amount of respiratory discomfort ranked on a pain scale of 1 to 10	Fluid overload	Notify supervisor immediately
Discomfort, bruising, and discoloration at the site	Document the patient's amount of pain ranked on a pain scale of 1 to 10; describe the color and measure the size of the area with discoloration	Hematoma	Notify supervisor immediately
Blood around the site	Document the approximate amount of blood	Hemorrhage	Apply pressure and call for help; do not leave patient
Patient has cyanosis, low blood pressure, weak pulse, discomfort along the vein, unconsciousness	Document the patient's blood pressure and pulse; document the patient's amount of pain ranked on a pain scale of 1 to 10	Air embolus	Call for supervisor immediately; do not leave patient

As you monitor patients on IV therapy, many of the problems you encounter have the same signs and symptoms. The most common problems are

- Container is empty
- Solution is infusing faster or slower than scheduled
- Site is red, sore, or swollen
- Tubing is disconnected or leaking
- Needle is out of place

Of these problems, the one you will see most frequently is a slow infusion. Recall from Chapter 6 that several factors may cause the slowing of an IV infusion:

- The solution bag is lower than 36 inches (1 meter) above the IV site
- The IV site has been taped too tightly
- The clamp on the tubing is closed
- The tubing is kinked, especially right above the bulb attached to the needle at the Y injection site
- The gauge of the catheter is too small to accommodate the fluid being infused
- Blood has backed up in the tubing
- The line contains air bubbles
- The patient has bent the elbow or wrist where the IV is inserted
- The IV has become interstitial, which means that the IV fluid is leaking into the tissue around the blood vessel

If you encounter an IV that is sluggish or has stopped, check for any of the problems just listed. Unkink the tubing or open the clamp if these actions are within your scope of practice. When troubleshooting an IV problem, consult with a more-experienced colleague who may see something that you overlooked. If the cause cannot be identified or resolved, the IV may need to be discontinued and restarted at another site. Once a problem is corrected, document your actions. Remember, if it is not documented, it is not done.

Patient Education & Communication

Keep the Patient Informed

When you are troubleshooting an IV, always keep your patient informed so as not to cause undue concern. If you cannot salvage the site and must establish a new access, communicate this information to your patient and provide any necessary patient education.

Checkpoint Questions 7-3

1. You find an IV site that is swollen and painful, and the patient has a temperature. What do you document?

_____

_____

2. If you cannot correct a problem with a slowed or stopped IV infusion, what should you do?

_____

_____

Before you continue to the next section, answer the previous Checkpoint Questions and complete the Monitoring IV Therapy activity under Chapter 7 on the student CD.

7-4 Documenting Fluid Balance

As you learned in Chapter 1, in an adult weighing 155 lb (70 kg), about 60 percent of the total body weight is fluid. In an infant, fluids account for about 80 percent of the total body weight. The body's fluid balance is regulated by hormones and is affected by fluid volume, by distribution of fluids in the body, and by the concentration of solutes in the fluid itself. Each day, the body gains fluids naturally by oral intake (liquids and water in foods) and respiration. It loses fluids naturally through respiration, perspiration, urine, and feces. Gains must equal losses to maintain the body's daily fluid balance.

Most adult patients should take in 1500 to 2000 mL of fluid per day. Fluid intake and fluid output do not need to be exactly equal, but the totals should be within 200 to 300 mL of each other for every 24-hour period. If this natural balance of fluids cannot be maintained because the patient is ill and unable to replace lost fluids orally, the patient is given IV therapy. Once an IV is started, it becomes necessary to monitor the patient's fluid balance by documenting the fluids that the patient receives and loses. This documentation is called **intake and output (I&O)**.

Intake and Output

Intake is the measurement of all fluids taken in from any source; it includes oral fluids, fluid from IV infusion, and fluid from a nasogastric (NG) or gastric (G) tube. Any fluid or nutrient that is liquid at room temperature is counted as intake. Output is a measurement of urine, wound or tube drainage, diarrhea, and vomiting. Fluid is also lost through respiration and perspiration, although these losses can only be estimated and are not recorded.

Seriously ill patients—for example, patients with dehydration, shock, septicemia, or renal failure or patients who have just had surgery—require strict and accurate fluid balance monitoring. These patients may even require hourly intake and output measurements. Hourly urine measurements are accurately obtained with the use of a **urometer** (a specialized urine collection bag with a flow meter) (Figure 7-3). A strict record of each patient's output, IV infusion, and oral intake must be maintained for each 24-hour period.

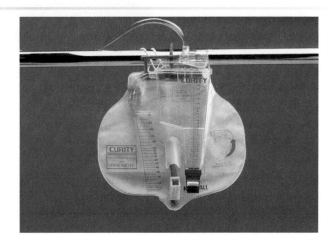

Figure 7-3 When a patient must have hourly intake and output recorded, a urometer as part of a urinary catheter can be used to measure the urine.

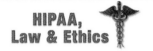
Patient Education & Communication

Ensuring Accurate Intake and Output

When intake and output recording is required during IV therapy, all measurements must be accurate. Stress to the patient as well as to the patient's family and visitors the importance of measuring the patient's intake and output. Provide education to family members who may feel that they are helping when they empty a urinal or bedpan. Instruct the patient to call you after using the bedpan or urinal so that you can measure the output amount. If the patient is ambulatory and able to use the toilet, instruct the patient to place the urine collection container under the toilet seat to collect the urine to be measured (Figure 7-4). Remind the patient and visitors that no one but the patient should drink from the water pitcher or consume fluids from the meal tray, that doing so could lead to erroneous information about the patient's fluid balance.

Figure 7-4 When a patient's intake and output is being recorded, you may need to collect and measure the urine in a collection hat placed under the toilet seat such as this one.

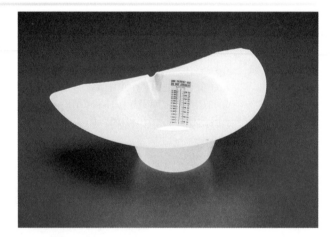

Documenting Fluids

Record intake and output on the patient's flow sheet or on an **intake and output (I&O) record** (Figure 7-5). The I&O record is often kept beside the patient's bed so that amounts can be easily recorded by any caregiver providing fluids or emptying bedpans, urinals, or emesis basins. Typically, the information on the flow sheet is transferred to the patient's medical chart at the end of each shift.

Figure 7-5 The intake and output record provides spaces for recording all of a patient's intake and output. It can be a paper form such as this one.

INTAKE/OUTPUT RECORD (SHIFT)

DATE	Shift	INTAKE (in mL's)						OUTPUT (in mL's)				
		Oral	Enteral NG/GT	Flush	IV	Enema	TOTAL	Urine	Emesis	BM	Other	TOTAL
	7–3											
	3–11											
	11–7											
24 Hour Total												
	7–3											
	3–11											
	11–7											
24 Hour Total												
	7–3											
	3–11											
	11–7											
24 Hour Total												
	7–3											
	3–11											
	11–7											
24 Hour Total												
	7–3											
	3–11											
	11–7											
24 Hour Total												
	7–3											
	3–11											
	11–7											
24 Hour Total												
	7–3											
	3–11											
	11–7											
24 Hour Total												

WEEKLY INTAKE AND OUTPUT EVALUATION

Average 24 Hour Intake: _____ ml

Average 24 Hour Output: _____ ml

Urine Color: _____

Urine Odor: ☐Normal ☐Strong ☐Foul

Skin Turgor: _____ Edema: _____

Consistency: ☐Normal ☐Thick

Clarity: ☐Clear ☐Cloudy ☐Sediment

Mucous Membrane: ☐Dry ☐Moist

Comments: _____

Evaluated By: (Signature/Title) _____ Date _____

Resident Name _____ ID # _____ Room # _____ Physician _____

I&O records may provide several spaces under the category "intravenous" to allow adequate room for charting on patients with more than one IV or more than one solution being infused. When documenting for these patients, ensure that each space on the I&O record is properly labeled with the correct solution.

When recording IV intake, you will document three amounts:

1. **IV to be absorbed (TBA)**—the amount of fluid in the solution container at the time you total the fluid balance record or at the end of your shift
2. **IV absorbed**—the total amount of fluid absorbed during your shift
3. **IV medication amounts**—the type and amount of fluid absorbed with intermittent medications infused during your shift

Document the IV absorbed at the end of your shift. This task is part of the shift report and is written on the intake and output record. In ICUs, emergency departments, and critical care units, recording of IV absorbed may be more frequent (Figure 7-6).

Document the time that the IV was started, The milliliters of fluid in the container when the IV was started, the amount of fluid remaining, and the IV absorbed. The amount of fluid remaining becomes the IV (TBA) for the next shift or the person taking over care of the patient. If the patient is on an infusion pump, record the total IV fluids infused (total milliliters), including any secondary fluids, at the end of your shift. The pump is cleared at the end of every shift.

A particular issue that frequently arises at the change of shift is an infusion that runs out before the next shift finishes report and begins to make patient rounds. Several actions can be taken to avoid this problem. When going off shift, do your IV tallies last so that amount remaining will be as accurate as possible. If the container has less than 100 mL, replace the container.

Figure 7-6 An electronic IV flow sheet tracks the types and amounts of fluid that a patient is receiving.

Mon. Sep. 6 12:42	Eclipsys Continuum	User: BISJAB1				

Login | Logout | Census | Patient | Config | Utility

Mail | Visits

Sections: Flowsheet | Notes | Medications | Labs I | Labs II | Review | Rehab

Forms: Vitals | 180 | Resp | Neuro | Wt & Meas | Interventn | Shft Assess | Pt History | 180 Summ | Withdrawal

180 Flowsheet

				09/06 09:00	10:00	11:00	12:00	13:00	15:00 Shift
T O T	**GRAND**	Total	Intake Output Net 24Hr	202.00 202.00 +504	382.00 220.00 162.00 +666	436.00 436.00 +1102	676.00 400.00 276.00 +1378	202.00 202.00 +504	1998.00 620.00 1378.00 +1378
	URINE	Urine	cc cc/kg cc/kg/hr		220.00				
	BLOOD	Blood Product Balance	Blood Prod. In Est. Blood Loss Net 24Hr		100.00 100.00 +180	180.00 180.00 +360			
I N	**CRYST**	05 WATER W/KCL & BICARB 200 ml/hr	o	200.00	200.00	200.00	200.00		1000.00
		IVPB Meds							
		KCL				50.00	50.00		100.00
	DRIPS	DSW-Versed 100mg/100ml 2.0 ml/hr	o	2.00	2.00	6.00	6.00		18.00
	BLOOD	Cryoprecipitate	24Hr						
		Fresh Frozen Plasma	24Hr		180.00 +180	180.00 +360	420.00 +780		780.00 +780
	ENTERAL	Water							
	DIET	Dietary Intake	Fluid Volume Solid Food						
O U T	**URINE**	Foley	24Hr		220.00 +220		400.00 +620		620.00 +620
		Urine	24Hr						
T E S T S	**STOOL**	Stool Count							

Whatever method you use for documentation, accuracy is of the utmost importance. If you do not document exact amounts, you are providing inaccurate information to the patient's health care team, and you may inadvertently cause inappropriate treatment for the patient.

Checkpoint Questions 7-4

1. When is an I&O record sheet required?

_____

_____

2. What is the difference between IV to be absorbed and IV absorbed?

_____

_____

Before you continue to the next section, answer the previous Checkpoint Questions and complete the Documenting Fluid Balance activity under Chapter 7 on the student CD.

7-5 Discontinuing an IV

An IV is discontinued when a patient no longer needs to receive IV therapy or when the access has been compromised and a new access needs to be initiated. This section describes the discontinuation procedure. Appendix F contains the competency checklist for discontinuing an IV; refer to this checklist if you are required to perform this skill in a laboratory or clinical situation.

To begin, gather the equipment: sterile 2×2 gauze pads, tape, and clean gloves. You will also need the patient's medical record and a method of recording the procedure. As with all procedures, start by washing your hands and putting on gloves to prevent infection and to follow Standard Precautions. Explain the procedure to the patient. Tell the patient that the procedure of removing the catheter is typically painless, but that removing the tape and dressing can cause some discomfort and tugging on the skin. Your explanation should alleviate the patient's concerns and gain his or her cooperation. Your next step is to turn off the infusion to prevent the IV from flowing after it is removed from the vein.

Loosen the dressing carefully without disturbing the catheter. Stabilize the catheter during the entire procedure to prevent trauma at the insertion site or injury to the vein (Figure 7-7). Ensure that the catheter is free, then place a piece of sterile 2×2 gauze over the site. Withdraw the catheter carefully and smoothly while simultaneously pressing down with the gauze to control bleeding. However, do not put pressure on the catheter while it is still in the vein. During the withdrawal, keep the catheter almost flush with the skin. This action should be swift, bloodless, and discrete. If the patient is excitable or apprehensive, distract his or her gaze and attention momentarily while you quickly and smoothly withdraw the cannula.

Immediately press the sterile 2×2 gauze over the site. Either you or your patient can apply steady pressure for up to 2 to 3 minutes or until the bleeding stops. A longer period of pressure may be required if the patient

Figure 7-7 When removing the dressing, stabilize the catheter to prevent bleeding or injury to the vein. In this picture the left hand is holding the catheter tip in place while the right hand is removing the tape from the IV site.

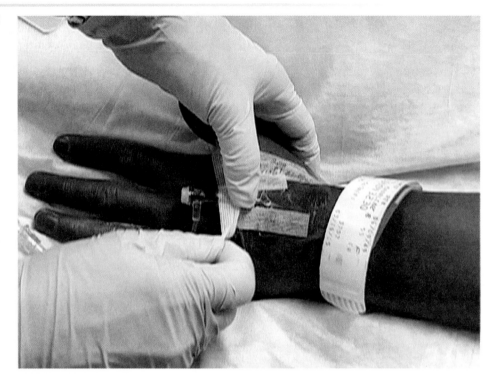

has received **anticoagulants** (blood thinners), had a large-gauge catheter, or has marked hypertension.

Remove the gauze pad and replace it with a clean, sterile gauze pad and tape or a Band-Aid. Elevate the arm to reduce venous pressure and facilitate clot formation. Instruct the patient to not flex the muscle at the insertion site. Flexing may increase the size of the wound in the vessel wall, which may cause additional bleeding and bruising.

If the catheter does not need to be sent to the lab for culture, you can remove your gloves while covering the catheter tip and place the catheter in a biohazardous waste container (Figure 7-8). Observe the insertion site for

Figure 7-8 If the catheter tip does not need to be sent to the lab, you can dispose of it promptly by removing your gloves while covering the tip. Since the catheter tip is not a sharp, you can dispose of the glove and tip in a biohazardous waste container.

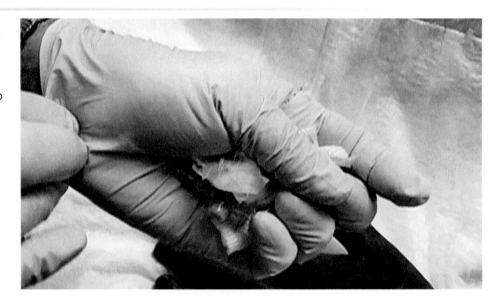

redness, swelling, and bleeding. Apply warm compresses if the site appears inflamed or irritated and if your facility's policy allows it.

Clean the area, and dispose of supplies and equipment properly. Make note of the amount of fluid that is left in the IV bag. Wash your hands, and record the volume infused in the I&O record. Ask the patient to report if the site begins to bleed again. In about 15 minutes, check the site again for bleeding or a hematoma.

When you document the procedure, remember to include the date, the time, the patient's response, the condition of the catheter, and your signature or initials. Here is an example of proper documentation: "10/04/07 10:30 IV discontinued from left hand—catheter intact. Denies pain. No swelling or bleeding noted at site. S. Sanchez LPN."

Safety and Infection Control

Preventing Bleeding

If your patient is receiving aspirin, warfarin (Coumadin), or heparin therapy, the IV site will have a greater tendency to bleed or develop a hematoma. After discontinuation of an IV infusion, maintain pressure on the venipuncture site for as long as necessary to prevent these complications.

Checkpoint Questions 7-5

1. How long should you apply pressure to the insertion site after you have discontinued an IV?

   _____

   _____

2. Why is it necessary to keep the catheter stabilized while you remove the tape when you discontinue an IV?

   _____

   _____

Before you continue to the chapter summary, answer the previous Checkpoint Questions and complete the Discontinuing an IV activity under Chapter 7 on the student CD.

Chapter Summary

- Documentation of IV therapy must occur after initiation of an IV, during the course of therapy, and on discontinuation.
- Documentation always includes the date, the time, and the name of the person performing the procedure. Additional information about the catheter, the IV site, and the patient's condition are also documented throughout IV therapy.
- Ambiguous terms and abbreviations should never be used in the documentation of IV therapy. Guidelines for appropriate abbreviations are established by JCAHO and by each health care facility.

- Patients on IV therapy must be monitored regularly. Documentation includes the amount and type of IV fluids administered, other fluid intake and output, any signs or symptoms of fluid deficit or excess, any signs and symptoms of sodium and potassium deficit or excess.
- Patients on IV therapy must have their fluid intake and output recorded so fluid balance can be maintained. Oral fluid intake, IV infusions, and tube feeding are recorded as intake. Urine, diarrhea, vomiting, and drainage are recorded as output.
- *IV absorbed* is the total amount of fluid absorbed by a patient during a shift. *IV to be absorbed (TBA)* is the amount of fluid left in the solution container at the end of a shift or at the time the fluid balance record is totaled.
- Precautions to be taken during IV discontinuation include maintaining Standard Precautions, stabilizing the catheter while removing the tape, and keeping pressure on the site after removal to stop any bleeding and prevent a hematoma.
- IV discontinuation documentation includes the date and time that the IV was discontinued, the condition of the catheter, the patient's response, whether an arm board was used, and whether the catheter was sent to the lab.

Multiple Choice

1. Documentation recommendations for IV fluids include which of the following?
   a. Electrolyte imbalance, fluid deficit and excess, fluid intake and output, solution composition
   b. Electrolyte imbalance, fluid deficit and excess, fluid intake and output, solution volume
   c. Electrolyte imbalance, fluid deficit and excess, fluid intake and output, solution volume and composition
   d. Electrolyte imbalance, fluid deficit and excess, fluid intake and output, solution volume, laboratory serum electrolyte values

2. Which of the following would be the most appropriate response if a patient asks, "Will it hurt when you remove the IV?"
   a. "No, not at all. It only hurts when it is inserted."
   b. "It will definitely hurt when I pull off the tape."
   c. "You will have pain, so I plan to give you a local anesthetic before I begin."
   d. "You may feel some discomfort and tugging when I remove the tape."

3. Which of the following medications would *not* be a consideration when you discontinue an IV?
   a. aspirin
   b. acetaminophen
   c. Coumadin
   d. heparin

4. Which of the following items is *not* typically documented when you discontinue an IV?
   a. the condition of the IV site
   b. the patient's response
   c. the size of the catheter
   d. the condition of the catheter

5. Which of the following items is *not* typically documented when you initiate an IV?
   a. the location of the IV site
   b. the patient's response
   c. the size of the catheter
   d. the condition of the catheter

6. The amount of fluid left in the solution container at the time you total the fluid balance record or at the end of your shift is called the
   a. IV (TBA).
   b. IV.
   c. IV absorbed.
   d. total intake.

7. The total amount of fluid absorbed on your shift is called the
   a. IV (TBA).
   b. IV.
   c. IV absorbed.
   d. total intake.

8. Which of the following should be documented as intake on the patient's record?
   a. The patient eats some crackers.
   b. An IV medication is hung as a secondary fluid.
   c. The catheter is irrigated with 60 mL of normal saline and is withdrawn.
   d. The patient is breathing rapidly.

9. When preparing to discontinue an IV, you would first
   a. turn off the IV infusion.
   b. quickly remove all the tape.
   c. put on a mask.
   d. moisten the transparent dressing with alcohol.

10. If a registered nurse initiated an IV, who should document the procedure?
    a. the medical assistant
    b. the LPN or LVN
    c. the registered nurse
    d. an administrative assistant

11. Which of the following is counted as intake?
    a. crackers
    b. drainage
    c. urine
    d. D5W

Matching

Match the correct documentation with the associated complication.

_____ 12. respiratory rate, blood pressure, and pain scale   a. infection

_____ 13. pain scale, and size and area of discoloration   b. infiltration

_____ 14. temperature, pain scale, and amount   c. fluid overload
         of swelling at site   d. air embolus

_____ 15. blood pressure, pulse, and pain scale   e. hematoma

_____ 16. coolness of skin, pain scale, and IV flow rate

Fill-in-the-Blank

17. When discontinuing an IV, apply steady pressure up to 2 to 3 minutes. Longer time may be needed if the patient is taking _____ .

18. Your patient has complaints of difficult breathing and rapid respirations and has been profusely diaphoretic for 3 days. You are concerned about his fluid balance because you know that these symptoms can mean that the patient is experiencing _____ .

19. Standards for intravenous therapy have been set by _____ .

20. If a patient exhibits signs of infection when you remove the IV, the _____ should be cut with sterile scissors and sent to the lab to be cultured.

21. Urine, diarrhea, and drainage are all considered part of a patient's _____ .

True/False

T   F   **22.** The abbreviation "MS" should be used when the medication morphine sulfate is administered.

T   F   **23.** The exact location of each attempt and the final successful site of an IV should always be documented.

T   F   **24.** If an infection is suspected, you should always take and document the patient's temperature.

T   F   **25.** Patient education is not included in documentation of IV therapy.

T   F   **26.** Intake and output are always monitored when a patient is receiving IV therapy.

What Should You Do? (Critical Thinking/Application Questions)

1. As part of your patient education for a patient on aspirin therapy, when you discontinue her IV you instruct her to apply pressure to the site and to not flex her arm. The patient questions your instructions. How would you explain the importance of these actions?

_____

_____

_____

Get Connected

Visit the McGraw-Hill Higher Education website for *Intravenous Therapy for Health Care Personnel* at **www.mhhe.com/healthcareskills** to complete the following activity.

1. The Joint Commission on Accreditation of Healthcare Organizations provides information and standards on their website related to IV therapy and documentation. Search for information about abbreviations that should not be used in documentation. Search also for guidelines to help health care facilities establish policies for infusion therapy.

Using the Student CD

Now that you have completed the material in Chapter 7, return to the student CD and complete any chapter activities you have not yet done. Practice your terminology with the Key Term Concentration game. Review the chapter material with the Spin the Wheel game. Take the final chapter test, complete the troubleshooting question, and e-mail or print your results to document your proficiency for this chapter.

8 Intravenous Therapy Calculations

Chapter Outline

I. Introduction
II. Calculating Flow Rates
   a. Calculating Flow Rates in Milliliters per Hour (mL/h)
      i. Using the Formula Method
      ii. Using Dimensional Analysis
   b. Calculating Flow Rates in Drops per Minute (gtt/min)
      i. Using the Formula Method
      ii. Using Dimensional Analysis
III. Adjusting Flow Rates
IV. Calculating Infusion Time and Volume
   a. Calculating Infusion Time
      i. Using the Formula Method
      ii. Using Dimensional Analysis
   b. Calculating Infusion Volume
      i. Using the Formula Method
      ii. Using Dimensional Analysis
V. Calculating Intermittent Infusions
   a. Secondary Lines (Piggyback)
   b. Intermittent Peripheral Infusion Devices
   c. Preparing and Calculating Intermittent Infusions

Learning Outcomes

- Calculate the flow rate for electronic infusion devices and manually controlled IV infusions.
- Adjust the flow rate for IV infusions.
- Calculate the infusion time based on volume and flow rate.
- Calculate the volume based on infusion time and flow rate.
- Calculate the amount to administer for intermittent IV infusion medications.

Key Terms

amount to administer (*A*)
calibration factor (*C*)
desired dose (*D*)
dosage unit (*Q*)
dose on hand (*H*)
drop factor
gtt/min

intermittent peripheral infusion device
IVPB
macrodrip
microdrip
mL/h

8-1 Introduction

IV fluids, additives, and medications must be administered with accuracy. There is a desperate need to avoid errors in order to prevent patient complications. To properly administer an IV infusion, you must know the flow rate in milliliters per hour and/or drops per minute. You should be able to calculate the infusion time and volume. You also need to know how to calculate a medication that is to be administered on an intermittent basis. Never administer an IV to a patient until you know the exact information about the amount, rate, and time. When an IV is ordered, you calculate the amount, rate, and time; then you monitor the infusion; and finally, you document the results.

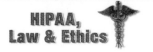

Checkpoint Question 8-1

1. What information must you calculate to administer IV fluids, additives, and medications?

   _____

   _____

If you are feeling a little rusty about your basic math skills, complete the Basic Math Review activity under Chapter 8 on the student CD before you continue to the next section.

HIPAA, Law & Ethics

Preventing Malpractice

When calculating IV flow rates and medications, accuracy is essential. An inaccurate rate or dose can cause severe consequences to the patient and possibly lead to medical malpractice. Remember, if you are not sure about your calculation, double-check yourself and/or ask for assistance.

8-2 Calculating Flow Rates

A physician's order for IV therapy indicates the amount of an IV fluid to be administered and the length of time over which it is to be given. Before you administer an IV, use these two values to calculate the flow rate for the IV solution. The flow rate is calculated in milliliters per hour (**mL/h**) or drops per minute (**gtt/min**).

The flow rate in milliliters per hour is the most common number that you must calculate. You need this information to set most electronic infusion devices. The flow rate in drops per minute is calculated when no pump is used or when you want to check the functioning of the electronic infusion device.

Calculating Flow Rates in Milliliters per Hour (mL/h)

Most electronic devices that regulate the flow of IV solutions will express the flow rate in milliliters per hour. You can use either a formula or dimensional analysis to calculate this rate. Before you begin, you must obtain the following information from the order for the IV:

- Volume (V), or amount to be administered, expressed in milliliters
- Time (T), expressed in hours (convert when necessary)

You will then calculate the flow rate (F), to be rounded to the nearest tenth.

Using the Formula Method

Use the formula

$$F = \frac{V}{T}$$

to calculate the flow rate in milliliters per hour.

EXAMPLE 1

Find the flow rate.

Ordered: 500 mg ampicillin in 100 mL NS to infuse over 30 minutes

Solution:

In this example, the volume is expressed in milliliters, so $V = 100$ mL. Because the time is expressed in minutes, you must first convert 30 minutes to hours in order to find T. To convert minutes to hours, divide by 60:

$$30 \text{ min} \div 60 = 0.5 \text{ h}$$

You now have the necessary information in the proper units:

$$V = 100 \text{ mL}$$

$$T = 0.5 \text{ h}$$

Use the formula $F = \dfrac{V}{T}$

$$F = \frac{100 \text{ mL}}{0.5 \text{ h}}$$

$$F = 200 \text{ mL/h}$$

EXAMPLE 2

Find the flow rate.

Ordered: 500 mL 5% D 0.45% NS over 3 hours

Solution:

In this example, the units are already expressed in milliliters and hours:

$V = 500$ mL

$T = 3$ h

Use the formula $F = \dfrac{V}{T}$

$$F = \frac{500 \text{ mL}}{3 \text{ h}}$$

$F = 166.7$ mL/h

Round to the nearest whole number:

$F = 167$ mL/h

Using Dimensional Analysis

EXAMPLE 1

Find the flow rate.

Ordered: 500 mg ampicillin in 100 mL NS to infuse over 30 minutes

Solution:

1. Determine the units of measure for the answer (F) and place it as the unknown on one side of the equation:

   F mL/h =

2. On the right side of the equation, write a factor with the number of milliliters to be administered (V) on top and the length of time to be administered (T) on the bottom:

   $$F \text{ mL/h} = \frac{100 \text{ mL}}{30 \text{ min}}$$

3. Multiply by a second factor to convert the minutes to hours and place minutes in the numerator:

   $$F \text{ mL/h} = \frac{100 \text{ mL}}{30 \text{ min}} \times \frac{60 \text{ min}}{1 \text{ h}}$$

4. Cancel units on the right side of the equation. The remaining unit of measure on the right side of the equation should match the unknown unit of measure on the left side of the equation:

$$F \text{ mL/h} = \frac{100 \text{ mL}}{30 \text{ min}} \times \frac{60 \text{ min}}{1 \text{ h}}$$

5. Solve the equation:

$$F \text{ mL/h} = \frac{100 \times 60}{30}$$

$$F = 200 \text{ mL/h}$$

EXAMPLE 2

Find the flow rate.

Ordered: 500 mL 5% D 0.45%S over 3 hours

Solution:

1. Determine the units of measure for the answer (*F*) and place it as the unknown on one side of the equation:

$$F \text{ mL/h} =$$

2. On the right side of the equation, write a factor with the number of milliliters to be administered (*V*) on top and the length of time to be administered (*T*) on the bottom:

$$F \text{ mL/h} = \frac{500 \text{ mL}}{3 \text{ h}}$$

3. Because the units of measurement on the left side of the equation match the units of measurement on the right side of the equation, no additional conversion factors are necessary. Solve the equation:

$$F \text{ mL/h} = \frac{500 \text{ mL}}{3 \text{ h}}$$

$$F = 166.7 \text{ mL/h}$$

4. Round to the nearest whole number:

$$F = 167 \text{ mL/h}$$

Calculating Flow Rates in Drops per Minute (gtt/min)

The flow rate for a manually regulated IV is calculated as the number of drops per minute. Before you can perform this calculation, you must first know how many drops are in a milliliter (as discussed in Chapter 3). IV tubing packages are labeled with a **drop factor,** which tells you how many drops of IV solution are equal to 1 mL when you use that tubing. **Macrodrip** tubing has larger drops and, typically, one of three drop factors: 10 gtt/mL, 15 gtt/mL, or 20 gtt/mL. **Microdrip** tubing has a drop factor of 60 gtt/mL (Figure 8-1).

In most circumstances, you will first determine the flow rate in milliliters per hour and then convert it to drops per minute. For example, you may need to manually check an electronic infusion device in order to monitor the flow rate of an IV. These devices usually express the flow rate in milliliters per hour. To check this device, you must convert the flow rate from milliliters per hour to drops per minute in order to count the drops delivered to the patient in a minute. To alter the flow rate of an IV *that is not attached to an electronic device,* adjust the roller or screw clamp so that the drops fall at the desired rate.

To determine the flow rate (f) in drops per minute, you must first determine the following:

- F, or the flow rate, expressed in milliliters per hour
- C, or the **calibration factor** of the tubing in drops per milliliter

Figure 8-1 Macrodrip tubing has a calibration factor of 10 gtt/mL, 15 gtt/mL, or 20 gtt/mL; microdrip tubing has a calibration of 60 gtt/mL.

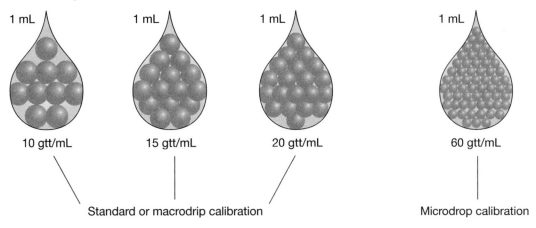

Using the Formula Method

To change the flow rate from milliliters per hour (F) to drops per minute (f), use the formula

$$f = \frac{F \times C}{60 \text{ min/hr}}$$

EXAMPLE 1

Find the flow rate in drops per minute that is equal to 75 mL/h when using 20 gtt/mL macrodrop tubing.

Solution:

$$F = 75 \text{ mL/h}$$

$$C = 20 \text{ gtt/mL}$$

Use the formula

$$f = \frac{F \times C}{60 \text{ min/hr}}$$

$$f = \frac{75 \text{ mL/h} \times 20 \text{ gtt/mL}}{60 \text{ min/h}}$$

Cancel the units:

$$f = \frac{75 \text{ m\cancel{L}/\cancel{h}} \times 20 \text{ gtt/m\cancel{L}}}{60 \text{ min/\cancel{h}}}$$

Solve the equation:

$$f = \frac{75 \times 20 \text{ gtt}}{60 \text{ min}}$$

$$f = 25 \text{ gtt/min}$$

EXAMPLE 2

Find the flow rate in drops per minute that is equal to 35 mL/h when using 60 gtt/mL microdrop tubing.

Solution:

$$F = 35 \text{ mL/h}$$

$$C = 60 \text{ gtt/mL}$$

Use the formula

$$f = \frac{F \times C}{60 \text{ min/hr}}$$

$$f = \frac{35 \text{ mL/h} \times 60 \text{ gtt/mL}}{60 \text{ min/h}}$$

Cancel the units:

$$f = \frac{35 \text{ m\cancel{L}/\cancel{h}} \times 60 \text{ gtt/m\cancel{L}}}{60 \text{ min/\cancel{h}}}$$

Solve the equation:

$$f = 35 \text{ gtt/min}$$

Notice that when microdrop tubing is used, the flow rate in drops per minute is the same as the flow rate in milliliters per hour. In other words, for 60 gtt/min microdrop tubing, $F = f$.

Using Dimensional Analysis

You can use dimensional analysis for calculating the flow rate in drops per minute by adding the drop factor of your tubing to the equation used for determining the flow rate in milliliters per hour.

EXAMPLE 1

Find the flow rate in drops per minute that is equal to 75 mL/h when using 20 gtt/mL macrodrop tubing.

Solution:

1. Determine the units of measure for the answer (f) and place it as the unknown on one side of the equation:

$$f \text{ gtt/min} =$$

2. On the right side of the equation, write a factor with the number of milliliters to be administered (V) on top and the length of time to be administered (T) on the bottom:

$$f \text{ gtt/min} = \frac{75 \text{ mL}}{h}$$

3. Multiply by a second factor to convert the hours to minutes and place the hour in the numerator:

$$f \text{ gtt/min} = \frac{75 \text{ mL}}{h} \times \frac{1 \text{ h}}{60 \text{ min}}$$

4. Multiply by the drop factor of the tubing being used:

$$f \text{ gtt/min} = \frac{75 \text{ mL}}{h} \times \frac{1 \text{ h}}{60 \text{ min}} \times \frac{20 \text{ gtt}}{1 \text{ mL}}$$

5. Cancel units on the right side of the equation. The remaining unit of measure on the right side of the equation should match the unknown unit of measure on the left side of the equation. (If not, check your equation.)

$$f \text{ gtt/min} = \frac{75 \text{ m\cancel{L}}}{\cancel{h}} \times \frac{1 \text{ \cancel{h}}}{60 \text{ min}} \times \frac{20 \text{ gtt}}{1 \text{ m\cancel{L}}}$$

6. Solve the equation:

$$f = \frac{75 \times 20 \text{ gtt}}{60 \text{ min}}$$

$$f = 25 \text{ gtt/min}$$

EXAMPLE 2

Find the flow rate in drops per minute that is equal to 35 mL/h when using 60 gtt/mL microdrop tubing.

Solution:

1. Determine the units of measure for the answer (f) and place it as the unknown on one side of the equation:

$$f \text{ gtt/min} =$$

2. On the right side of the equation, write a factor with the number of milliliters to be administered (V) on top and the length of time to be administered (T) on the bottom:

$$f \text{ gtt/min} = \frac{35 \text{ mL}}{h}$$

3. Multiply by a second factor to convert the hours to minutes and place the hour in the numerator:

$$f \text{ gtt/min} = \frac{35 \text{ mL}}{h} \times \frac{1 \text{ h}}{60 \text{ min}}$$

4. Multiply by the drop factor of the tubing being used:

$$f \text{ gtt/min} = \frac{35 \text{ mL}}{h} \times \frac{1 \text{ h}}{60 \text{ min}} \times \frac{60 \text{ gtt}}{1 \text{ mL}}$$

5. Cancel units on the right side of the equation. The remaining unit of measure on the right side of the equation should match the unknown unit of measure on the left side of the equation. (If not, check your equation.)

$$f \text{ gtt/min} = \frac{35 \text{ m\cancel{L}}}{\cancel{h}} \times \frac{1 \text{ \cancel{h}}}{60 \text{ min}} \times \frac{60 \text{ gtt}}{1 \text{ m\cancel{L}}}$$

6. Solve the equation:

$$f \text{ gtt/min} = \frac{35 \times 1 \times \cancel{60} \text{ gtt}}{\cancel{60} \text{ min}}$$

$$f = 35 \text{ gtt/min}$$

Notice that the tubing factor of 60 gtt/min cancels the time factor of 1h over 60 min. For microdrop tubing, the additional step of multiplying by the drop factor is not necessary.

Checkpoint Question 8-2

1. Determine the flow rate in milliliters per hour and drops per minute for the following order:

   500 mL LR IV q8h using tubing calibrated at 15 gtt/mL

   _____

   _____

Before you continue to the next section, answer the previous Checkpoint Question and complete the Calculating Flow Rates activity under Chapter 8 on the student CD.

8-3 Adjusting Flow Rates

Drop counting and timing are not always precise. What you calculate to be 25 drops per minute may actually be 25.4 drops per minute. Additionally, no matter how accurate an electronic infusion device may appear to be, it must be checked to ensure that the IV is flowing at the proper rate. Adjustments to flow rates sometimes need to be made. You should check at least once every hour to see if an IV is infusing behind or ahead of schedule. Your facility's policy will dictate whether you may adjust the IV flow rate or whether you should notify the physician. Always check this policy before adjusting a flow rate.

To adjust the flow rate, you will need to recalculate the infusion using the volume (*V*) remaining in the IV, the time (*T*) remaining in the order, and the calibration factor (*C*) of the tubing.

EXAMPLE 1

Original order: 1500 mL NS over 12 hours (This is a flow rate of 125 mL/h)
The IV was infused at an original rate of 42 gtt/min using 20 gtt/mL macrodrop tubing.
After 3 hours, 1200 mL remain in the bag (3 × 125 = 375 mL should have been infused).
Facility policy: flow rate adjustments must not exceed 25 percent.

Solution:

$$V = 1200 \text{ mL (volume remaining)}$$

$$T = 9 \text{ h (original 12 hours minus the elapsed 3 hours)}$$

$$C = 20 \text{ gtt/mL (calibration of the tubing)}$$

Because the time is expressed in hours, you must first convert 9 hours to minutes in order to find *T*. To convert hours to minutes, multiply by 60:

$$9 \text{ h} \times 60 = 540 \text{ min}$$

Use the formula

$$f = C \times \frac{V}{T}$$

$$f = 20 \text{ gtt/mL} \times \frac{1200 \text{ mL}}{540 \text{ min}}$$

Cancel the units:

$$f = 20 \text{ gtt/m\cancel{L}} \times \frac{1200 \text{ m\cancel{L}}}{540 \text{ min}}$$

Solve the equation:

$$f = 20 \text{ gtt} \times \frac{1200}{540 \text{ min}}$$

$$f = 44.4 \text{ gtt/min}$$

Round to the nearest whole number:

$$f = 44 \text{ gtt/min}$$

The adjusted flow rate is 44 drops per minute. Now you must determine whether the adjusted flow rate is within the facility policy of 25 percent. Multiply the original flow rate of 42 drops per minute by 25:

$$42 \times 25\% = 10.5$$

The adjusted rate must fall within the following range:

$$42 - 10.5 = 31.5 \text{ gtt/min minimum}$$

$$42 + 10.5 = 52.5 \text{ gtt/min maximum}$$

Because 44 drops per minute falls between the minimum and maximum allowed by the policy, you may adjust the rate.

EXAMPLE 2

Original order: 1500 mL NS over 12 hours (original flow rate in mL/h = 125)

The IV was infused at an original rate of 30 gtt/min using 15 gtt/mL macrodrop tubing.

After 4 hours, 1100 mL remain in the bag. (400 mL have infused. 500 mL should have infused)

Facility policy: flow rate adjustments must not exceed 25 percent.

Solution:

$$V = 1100 \text{ mL}$$

$$T = 8 \text{ h } (12 \text{ hr} - 4 \text{ hr})$$

$$C = 15 \text{ gtt/mL}$$

Convert hours to minutes:

$$8 \text{ h} \times 60 = 480 \text{ min}$$

Use the formula

$$f = C \times \frac{V}{T}$$

$$f = 15 \text{ gtt/mL} \times \frac{1100 \text{ mL}}{480 \text{ min}}$$

Cancel the units:

$$f = 15 \text{ gtt/}\cancel{mL} \times \frac{1100 \; \cancel{mL}}{480 \text{ min}}$$

Solve the equation:

$$f = 15 \text{ gtt} \times \frac{1100}{480 \text{ min}}$$

$$f = 34.4 \text{ gtt/min}$$

Round to the nearest whole number:

$$f = 34 \text{ gtt/min}$$

Determine if the adjusted rate is within facility policy:

$$30 \times 25\% = 7.5$$

$$30 - 7.5 = 22.5 \text{ gtt/min minimum}$$

$$30 + 7.5 = 37.5 \text{ gtt/min maximum}$$

Because 34 drops per minute falls between the minimum and maximum allowed by the policy, you may adjust the rate.

Troubleshooting Recalculating a Flow Rate

The physician's IV order for your patient is 750 mL D5NS to infuse over 8 h. You calculate that the patient should receive 94 mL per hour with a flow rate of 16 gtt/min using 10 gtt/mL tubing. After 4 hours you notice that 450 mL remain in the bag, and the patient is scheduled for a test in the next hour.

What should you do?

_____

_____

Patient Education & Communication Keep the Patient Informed

When you adjust the rate of an IV infusion, communicate to the patient what you are doing so as to not cause the patient any concern or confusion about his or her treatment.

Checkpoint Question 8-3

1. Calculate the original flow rate in milliliters per hour and drops per minute. Determine if an adjustment is necessary; if so, calculate the adjusted flow rate.

   Original order: 1000 mL RL over 8 hours (15 gtt/mL tubing)
   After 2 hours, 125 mL have infused

   _____

   _____

Before you continue to the next section, answer the previous Checkpoint Question and complete the Adjusting Flow Rates activity under Chapter 8 on the student CD.

8-4 Calculating Infusion Time and Volume

An order may call for a certain amount of fluid to infuse at a specific rate but does not specify the duration. In this situation, you need to calculate the duration, or amount of time the IV will take to infuse, so that you can monitor the IV properly. In other situations, you may know the duration and the flow rate but will need to calculate the fluid volume.

Calculating Infusion Time

To calculate infusion time in hours (T), you must first determine the following:

- Volume (V), expressed in milliliters
- Flow rate (F), expressed in milliliters per hour

You can use either a formula or dimensional analysis to calculate the time.

Using the Formula Method

Use the formula

$$T = \frac{V}{F}$$

to calculate the infusion time.

EXAMPLE 1

Find the total time to infuse.

Ordered: 1000 mL NS to infuse at a rate of 75 mL/h

Solution:

$$V = 1000 \text{ mL}$$

$$F = 75 \text{ mL/h}$$

Use the formula

$$T = \frac{V}{F}$$

$$T = \frac{1000 \text{ mL}}{75 \text{ mL/h}}$$

Cancel the units:

$$T = \frac{1000 \text{ m\cancel{L}}}{75 \text{ m\cancel{L}/h}}$$

Solve the equation:

$$T = \frac{1000}{75 \text{ h}}$$

$$T = 13.33 \text{ h}$$

Notice that 0.33 hours does not represent 33 minutes. You must multiply the fractional hours by 60 (the number of minutes in an hour) to convert the fraction to minutes:

$$0.33 \text{ h} \times 60 = 20 \text{ min}$$

The total time to infuse the solution is 13 hours and 20 minutes.

EXAMPLE 2

Find the total time to infuse.

Ordered: 750mL LR to infuse at a rate of 125 mL/h

Solution:

$$V = 750 \text{ mL}$$

$$F = 125 \text{ mL/h}$$

Use the formula

$$T = \frac{V}{F}$$

$$T = \frac{750 \text{ mL}}{125 \text{ mL/h}}$$

Cancel the units:

$$T = \frac{750 \text{ m\cancel{L}}}{125 \text{ m\cancel{L}/h}}$$

Solve the equation:

$$T = \frac{750}{125 \text{ h}}$$

$$T = 6 \text{ h}$$

The total time to infuse the solution is 6 hours.

Using Dimensional Analysis

EXAMPLE 1

Find the total time to infuse.

Ordered: 1000 mL NS to infuse at a rate of 75 mL/h

Solution:

1. Determine the units of measure for the answer (*T*) and place it as the unknown on one side of the equation:

    T h $=$

2. On the right side of the equation, write a factor with the number of milliliters to be administered (*V*) on top and the flow rate (*F*) on the bottom.

$$T\ h = \frac{1000\ mL}{75\ mL/h}$$

3. Cancel units on the right side of the equation. The remaining unit of measure on the right side of the equation should match the unknown unit of measure on the left side of the equation:

$$T\ h = \frac{1000\ \cancel{mL}}{75\ \cancel{mL}/h}$$

4. Solve the equation:

$$T\ h = \frac{1000}{75\ h}$$

$$T = 13.33\ h$$

Notice that 0.33 hours does not represent 33 minutes. You must multiply the fractional hours by 60 (the number of minutes in an hour) to convert the fraction to minutes:

$$0.33\ h \times 60 = 20\ min$$

The total time to infuse the solution is 13 hours and 20 minutes.

EXAMPLE 2

Find the total time to infuse.

Ordered: 750 mL LR to infuse at a rate of 125 mL/h

Solution:

1. Determine the units of measure for the answer (*T*) and place it as the unknown on one side of the equation.

    T h $=$

2. On the right side of the equation, write a factor with the number of milliliters to be administered (*V*) on top and the flow rate (*F*) on the bottom:

$$T\ h = \frac{750\ mL}{125\ mL/h}$$

3. Cancel units on the right side of the equation. The remaining unit of measure on the right side of the equation should match the unknown unit of measure on the left side of the equation:

$$T \, h = \frac{750 \, \text{mL}}{125 \, \text{mL/h}}$$

4. Solve the equation:

$$T \, h = \frac{750}{125 \, h}$$

$$T = 6 \, h$$

The total time to infuse the solution is 6 hours.

In some situations, you will need to calculate the time at which an infusion will be completed. For this calculation, you must first know the total infusion time in hours and minutes. Then you will convert the infusion start time into military time, perform the calculation, and convert the military time answer back into hours and minutes (see Figure 8-2). Because each day is only 24 hours long, when your sum is greater than 2400 (midnight), you must start a new day by subtracting 2400. The time of completion in this situation will be the next calendar day.

Figure 8-2 Military time is based on a 24-h clock.

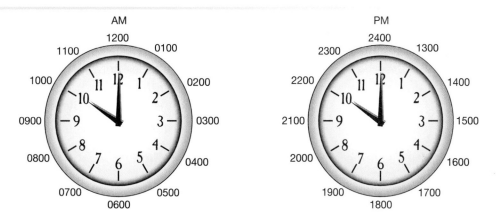

EXAMPLE 1

Determine when the following infusion will be completed.

Ordered: 1000 mL NS to infuse at a rate of 75 mL/h.
The infusion is started at 7 a.m. on 6/06/07.

Solution:

Determine the start time in military time:

7 a.m. = 0700

Add the total amount of time to infuse, which was determined earlier in Example 1 to be 13 hours and 20 minutes, or 1320:

0700 + 1320 = 2020

Convert military time to hours and minutes:

2020 = 8:20 p.m.

The solution should be infused by 8:20 p.m.

EXAMPLE 2

Determine when the following infusion will be completed.

Ordered: 750 mL LR to infuse at a rate of 125 mL/h.

The infusion is started at 11 p.m. on 8/04/07.

Solution:

Determine the start time in military time:

11 p.m. = 2300

Add the total amount of time to infuse, which was determined earlier in Example 2 to be 6 hours, or 0600:

2300 + 0600 = 2900

Because this total is greater than 2400 (the number of military hours in a day), subtract 2400 from the total:

2900 − 2400 = 500

Convert military time to hours and minutes:

0500 = 5 a.m.

The solution should be infused by 5 a.m. on 8/05/07.

Calculating Infusion Volume

To calculate infusion volume (V), you must first know the following:

- Time (T), expressed in hours
- Flow rate (F), expressed in milliliters per hour

You can use either a formula or dimensional analysis to calculate the volume.

Using the Formula Method

Use the formula

$$V = T \times F$$

to calculate the infusion volume.

EXAMPLE 1

Find the total volume infused or to be infused in 5 hours if the infusion rate is 35 mL/h.

Solution:

$T = 5$ h

$F = 35$ mL/h

Use the formula

$V = T \times F$

$V = 5$ h $\times 35$ mL/h

Solve the equation:

$V = 175$ mL

The total volume infused over 5 hours is 175 mL.

EXAMPLE 2

Find the total volume infused or to be infused in 12 hours if the infusion rate is 200 mL/h.

Solution:

$$T = 12\ h$$

$$F = 200\ mL/h$$

Use the formula

$$V = T \times F$$

$$V = 12\ h \times 200\ ml/h$$

Solve the equation:

$$V = 2400\ mL$$

The total volume infused over 12 hours is 2400 mL.

Using Dimensional Analysis

EXAMPLE 1

Find the total volume infused or to be infused in 5 hours if the infusion rate is 35 mL/h.

Solution:

1. Determine the units of measure for the answer (V) and place it as the unknown on one side of the equation:

$$V\ mL =$$

2. On the right side of the equation, write a factor with the length of time of the infusion (T) over 1:

$$V\ mL = \frac{5\ h}{1}$$

3. Multiply by the flow rate of the infusion (F):

$$V\ mL = \frac{5\ h}{1} \times \frac{35\ mL}{h}$$

4. Cancel units on the right side of the equation. The remaining unit of measure on the right side of the equation should match the unknown unit of measure on the left side of the equation:

$$V\ mL = \frac{5\ \cancel{h}}{1} \times \frac{35\ mL}{\cancel{h}}$$

5. Solve the equation:

$$V\ mL = \frac{5 \times 35}{1}$$

$$V = 175\ mL$$

The total volume infused over 5 hours is 175 mL.

EXAMPLE 2

Find the total volume infused or to be infused in 12 hours if the infusion rate is 200 mL/h.

Solution:

1. Determine the units of measure for the answer (V) and place it as the unknown on one side of the equation:

$$V \text{ mL} =$$

2. On the right side of the equation, write a factor with the length of time of the infusion (T) over 1:

$$V \text{ mL} = \frac{12 \text{ h}}{1}$$

3. Multiply by the flow rate of the infusion (F):

$$V \text{ mL} = \frac{12 \text{ h}}{1} \times \frac{200 \text{ mL}}{\text{h}}$$

4. Cancel units on the right side of the equation. The remaining unit of measure on the right side of the equation should match the unknown unit of measure on the left side of the equation:

$$V \text{ mL} = \frac{12 \cancel{\text{ h}}}{1} \times \frac{200 \text{ mL}}{\cancel{\text{h}}}$$

5. Solve the equation:

$$V \text{ mL} = \frac{12 \times 200}{1}$$

$$V = 2400 \text{ mL}$$

The total volume infused over 12 hours is 2400 mL.

Checkpoint Questions 8-4

1. Calculate the total time to infuse the following:
   Ordered: 1000 mL NS at 83 mL/h using an infusion pump

   _____

   _____

2. Determine when the following IV infusion will be completed.
   Ordered: 1500 mL D5W with 30 mEq KCL/L at a rate of 75 mL/h.
   You start the infusion at noon.

   _____

   _____

3. Find the total volume to administer. D5RL set at 100 mL/h for 8 h

   _____

   _____

Before you continue to the next section, answer the previous Checkpoint Questions and complete the Calculating Infusion Time and Volume activity under Chapter 8 on the student CD.

8-5 Calculating Intermittent Infusions

Intermittent infusion is most commonly used when a patient requires medications only at certain times. Intermittent medications can be delivered through a secondary IV line when the patient is receiving continuous IV therapy or a through a saline or heparin lock. When using a saline or heparin lock, utilize the same techniques as you would for an IV drip (pump or gravity drip). After you have administered the complete dose of medication, disconnect the tubing from the IV access device. Some medications are given by IV push, meaning that a syringe is connected to the IV access device and the medication is injected directly. IV push medications are usually injected slowly, especially those medications that might irritate the vein or that have an extremely rapid effect.

Secondary Lines (Piggyback)

A secondary administration set or line, also known as a *piggyback* or **IVPB,** is an IV setup that attaches to a primary administration set or line. It can be used to infuse medication or other compatible fluids on an intermittent basis, such as q6h (every 6 hours). Although shorter than primary tubing, secondary tubing has the same basic components. IVPB bags are smaller, often holding 50 mL, 100 mL, or 150 mL of fluid. The ADD-Vantage system from Abbott Laboratories is a secondary system (see Figure 8-3). It uses a specially designed IV bag into which you add medication directly from the vial, often in a powdered form. Any mixing takes place in the bag. The solution is then infused with the medication vial remaining in place.

Intermittent Peripheral Infusion Devices

You can administer medication to a patient on a regular, though not continuous, schedule by using an **intermittent peripheral infusion device.** These devices are more commonly known as heparin or saline locks. To create a

Figure 8-3 The ADD-Vantage system is an example of medication that is delivered through a secondary line.

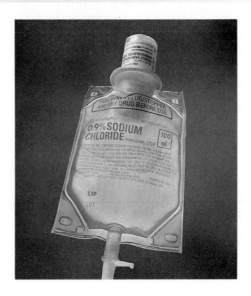

lock, attach an infusion port to an already-inserted IV catheter. This port allows you to infuse medication intermittently by injecting it directly into the vein using a secondary administration set. The physician's order will specify an IV piggyback for medications that are to be injected into an IV line or through a saline or heparin lock.

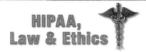

When a lock is used, fluids do not flow continuously through the IV needle or catheter. To prevent blockage of the line, flush the device two or three times a day or after administering medication. A saline lock is flushed or irrigated with saline. A heparin lock is flushed or irrigated with heparin solution, recall heparin is an anticoagulant that retards clot formation. The device used and the policy of your facility will dictate the amount and concentration of solution to use. Saline or heparin fills the infusion port and IV catheter, preventing blood from entering and becoming trapped. If blood were to become trapped, it would form a clot and block the catheter.

Preparing and Calculating Intermittent Infusions

Frequently, intermittent medications are already reconstituted and prepared for piggyback or for heparin or saline lock administration. In some situations, however, you may be required to reconstitute and prepare a medication for IV infusion or to calculate the amount to administer for an IV push medication. The flow rate for prepared medications is calculated in the same manner as regular IV infusions are, but the volume of fluid may be smaller, and the infusion time may be less than an hour. To calculate the flow rate, you may need to change minutes into hours.

When you administer an intermittent IV infusion through a saline or heparin lock, irrigate or flush the lock before or after administration. If you meet resistance when flushing a saline or heparin lock, stop the procedure immediately so that you do not force a clot into the bloodstream. Here are the steps to follow when you prepare medication for an intermittent IV infusion:

1. Reconstitute the medication using the label and package insert. Read the label and package insert carefully; use the correct type and amount of solution during reconstitution.
2. Calculate the amount to administer. For this calculation, you will first need to determine the following:
   - **Desired dose (D)**, or the amount of drug to be given at a single time
   - **Dosage unit (Q)**, or the unit by which the drug will be measured when administered
   - **Dose on hand (H)**, or the amount of drug contained in each dosage unit

With this information, you will be able to calculate the **amount to administer (A)**, or the volume of liquid that contains the desired dose.

3. Calculate the flow rate. You can use either a formula or dimensional analysis for this calculation.

EXAMPLE 1

Ordered: Eloxatin 75 mg in 250 mL D5W IV piggyback over 90 min
On hand: Eloxatin 100 mg (see the accompanying figures 8-4A and 8-4B)

Solution:

According to the package insert, Eloxatin should be reconstituted with 20 mL of water or 5% dextrose for injection. The dosage strength of the medication will be 100 mg/20 mL. Because the dosage ordered is 75 mg, you must calculate the amount to administer (A) by using the following information: desired dose (D), dose on hand (H), and dosage unit (Q). The formula that you use for this calculation is

$$A = \frac{D \times Q}{H}$$

The drug is ordered in milligrams, which is the same unit of measure as the dose on hand. You have the necessary information in the proper units:

$$D = 75 \text{ mg}$$

$$Q = 20 \text{ mL}$$

$$H = 100 \text{ mg}$$

Use the formula

$$A = \frac{D \times Q}{H}$$

$$A = \frac{75 \text{ mg} \times 20 \text{ mL}}{100 \text{ mg}}$$

Cancel the units:

$$A = \frac{75 \text{ m\!g} \times 20 \text{ mL}}{100 \text{ m\!g}}$$

Solve the equation:

$$A = \frac{75 \times 20 \text{ mL}}{100}$$

$$A = 15 \text{ mL}$$

The amount to administer is 15 mL.

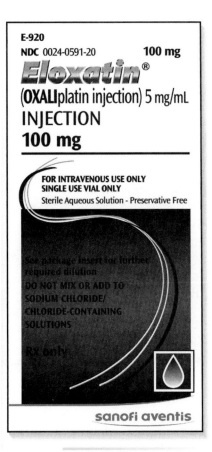

Figure 8-4A Always check the medication label before performing dosage calculations.

E-920
NDC 0024-0591-20   **100 mg**
Eloxatin®
(OXALIplatin injection**) 5 mg/mL**
INJECTION
100 mg

FOR INTRAVENOUS USE ONLY
SINGLE USE VIAL ONLY
Sterile Aqueous Solution - Preservative Free

See package insert for further
required dilution
DO NOT MIX OR ADD TO
SODIUM CHLORIDE/
CHLORIDE-CONTAINING
SOLUTIONS

Rx only

sanofi aventis

Figure 8-4B Always check the package insert before performing dosage calculations.

Dosage and Administration

Preparation of Infusion Solution

- ELOXATIN (oxaliplatin) IS NOT INTERCHANGEABLE WITH OTHER PLATINUMS. PLEASE VERIFY CORRECT DRUG AND DOSAGE PRIOR TO PREPARATION

- RECONSTITUTION OR FINAL DILUTION MUST NEVER BE PERFORMED WITH A SODIUM CHLORIDE SOLUTION OR OTHER CHLORIDE-CONTAINING SOLUTIONS

- The lyophilized powder is reconstituted by adding 10 mL (for the 50-mg vial) or 20 mL (for the 100-mg vial) of Water for Injection, USP, or 5% Dextrose Injection, USP

- **Do not administer the reconstituted solution without further dilution.**   The reconstituted solution must be further diluted in an infusion solution of 250-500 mL of 5% Dextrose Injection, USP

- After reconstitution in the original vial, the solution may be stored up to 24 hours under refrigeration (2-8°C [36-46°F])

- After final dilution with 250-500 mL of 5% Dextrose Injection, USP, the shelf life is **6 hours at room temperature (20-25°C [68-77°F]) or up to 24 hours under refrigeration (2-8°C [36-46°F])**

- ELOXATIN is not light sensitive

The package insert indicates that the reconstituted solution must be further diluted with an infusion solution of 250 to 500 mL of 5% dextrose injection, USP. The physician's order says to use 250 mL of D5W. Using a sterile needle and proper aseptic technique, withdraw 15 mL of the diluted solution and inject it into the 250-mL bag of D5W. Now you have a solution of 75 mg of Eloxatin in 250 D5W, which you must deliver over 90 minutes. Your next step is to calculate the flow rate in milliliters per hour.

Because the time is expressed in minutes, you must first convert 90 minutes to hours in order to find T. Remember that to convert minutes to hours, you divide by 60:

$$90 \text{ min} \div 60 = 1.5 \text{ h}$$

You now have the necessary information in the proper units:

$$V = 265 \text{ mL (250 mL of D5W and 15 mL of diluted medication)}$$

$$T = 1.5 \text{ h}$$

Use the formula $F = \dfrac{V}{T}$

$$F = \frac{265 \text{ mL}}{1.5 \text{ h}}$$

$$F = 176.6 \text{ mL/h}$$

Round to the nearest whole number:

$$F = 177 \text{ mL/h}$$

You would set the infusion pump to 177 mL/h.

If an infusion pump is not used, you will need to calculate the drops per minute. For this example, use standard tubing that is 15 gtt/mL. Always check the drop factor on the tubing packaging before doing your calculations. Remember that the formula for changing the flow rate from milliliters per hour (F) to drops per minute (f) is

$$f = \frac{F \times C}{60 \text{ min/hr}}$$

You have the necessary information in the proper units:

$$F = 177 \text{ mL/h}$$

$$C = 15 \text{ gtt/mL}$$

Use the formula

$$f = \frac{F \times C}{60 \text{ min/hr}}$$

$$f = \frac{177 \text{ mL/h} \times 15 \text{ gtt/mL}}{60 \text{ min/h}}$$

Cancel the units:

$$f = \frac{177 \text{ m\cancel{L}/\cancel{h}} \times 15 \text{ gtt/m\cancel{L}}}{60 \text{ min/\cancel{h}}}$$

Solve the equation:

$$f = \frac{177 \times 15 \text{ gtt}}{60 \text{ min}}$$

$$f = 44.25 \text{ gtt/min}$$

Round to the nearest whole number:

$$f = 44 \text{ gtt/min}$$

Safety and Infection Control

Preventing Errors

Ensure accurate calculations when administering IV medication and do not forget to follow the seven rights of medication administration including the right medication, the right patient, the right time, the right route, the right dose, the right technique, and the right documentation.

1. Determine the amount to administer and calculate the flow rate in milliliters per hour and drops per minute for the following:

Ordered: Fortaz 1.5 g IVPB over 30 min
On hand: (see the accompanying figure for the label, package insert, and IV tubing packaging 8-5A, 8-5B, 8-5C)

_____

_____

Before you continue to the chapter summary, answer the previous Checkpoint Question and complete the Intermittent Infusions activity under Chapter 8 on the student CD.

Figure 8-5A

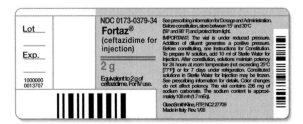

Figure 8-5C

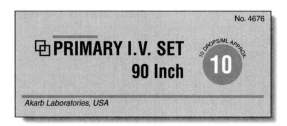

Figure 8-5B

All vials of FORTAZ as supplied are under reduced pressure. When FORTAZ is dissolved, carbon dioxide is released and a positive pressure develops. For ease of use please follow the recommended techniques of constitution described on the detachable Instructions for Constitution section of this insert.

Solutions of FORTAZ, like those of most beta-lactam antibiotics, should not be added to solutions of aminoglycoside antibiotics because of potential interaction.

However, if concurrent therapy with FORTAZ and an aminoglycoside is indicated, each of these antibiotics can be administered separately to the same patient.

Directions for Use of FORTAZ Frozen in Galaxy® Plastic Containers: FORTAZ supplied as a frozen, sterile, iso-osmotic, nonpyrogenic solution in plastic containers is to be administered after thawing either as a continuous or intermittent IV infusion. The thawed solution is stable for 24 hours at room temperature or for 7 days if stored under refrigeration. Do not refreeze.

Thaw container at room temperature (25°C) or under refrigeration (5°C). Do not force thaw by immersion in water baths or by microwave irradiation. Components of the solution may precipitate in the frozen state and will dissolve upon reaching room temperature with little or no agitation. Potency is not affected. Mix after solution has reached room temperature. Check for minute leaks by squeezing bag firmly. Discard bag if leaks are found as sterility may be impaired. Do not add supplementary medication. Do not use unless solution is clear and seal is intact.

Use sterile equipment.

Caution: Do not use plastic containers in series connections. Such use could result in air embolism due to residual air being drawn from the primary container before administration of the fluid from the secondary container is complete.

Preparation for Administration:
1. Suspend container from eyelet support.
2. Remove protector from outlet port at bottom of container.
3. Attach administration set. Refer to complete directions accompanying set.

Chapter Summary

- The flow rate for an electronic infusion device is calculated in milliliters per hour. For a manually controlled IV or when an electronic device needs to be checked, the flow rate is calculated in drops per minute.
- If the IV flow rate is too fast or too slow, it should be adjusted. The new flow rate is calculated from the amount of solution left in the bag and the time remaining for the infusion. The percentage or amount of adjustment is regulated by the facility; typically, the adjustment does not exceed 25 percent of the original flow rate.
- Sometimes the physician's order gives only the infusion rate and the volume of fluid to infuse. The duration, or amount of time the IV will take to infuse, must be calculated in order that the IV can be properly monitored.
- In some situations, the physician's order for an IV gives only the duration and the flow rate. For proper administration, the volume of fluid to be infused must be calculated.
- The three steps for administering intermittent medications are (1) reconstitute the medication, (2) calculate the amount to administer, and (3) calculate the flow rate.

Matching

_____ **1.** IVPB

_____ **2.** microdrip

_____ **3.** macrodrip

_____ **4.** drop factor

_____ **5.** mL/h

_____ **6.** gtt/min

a. number of drops needed to deliver 1 mL of fluid through IV tubing

b. the flow rate value for manually controlled IV infusions

c. administration of IV medications or fluids through a secondary line

d. IV tubing that delivers 10 gtt/mL, 15 gtt/mL or 20 gtt/mL

e. IV tubing that delivers 60 gtt/mL

f. flow rate value for most electronically controlled IVs

True/False

T   F   **7.** IV flow rates typically can be adjusted to within 25 percent of the original rate.

T   F   **8.** IV flow rates should always be adjusted so that the amount infused is caught back up within 2 hours.

T   F   **9.** Intermittent peripheral infusion devices include the IVPB and the secondary set.

T   F   **10.** To calculate the flow rate in milliliters per hour, divide the total volume by the number of hours for the infusion.

T   F   **11.** To determine the number of minutes in an hour, multiply by 60.

Multiple Choice

12. Ordered: 1000 mL LR over 6 h. What is the flow rate in milliliters per hour?
   a. 166.6 gtt/min
   b. 167 mL/h
   c. 167 gtt/min
   d. 166.6 mL/h

13. Ordered: 1000 mL NS over 24 h (20 gtt/mL tubing). What is the flow rate in drops per minute?
   a. 14 mL/h
   b. 42 mL/h
   c. 14 gtt/min
   d. 42 gtt/min

14. Ordered: 250 mL D5W over 3 h by infusion pump. What is the flow rate?
    a. 83 gtt/min
    b. 84 mL/h
    c. 83.3 mL/h
    d. 83 mL/h

15. Ordered: 500 mL LR at 125 mL/h using microdrip tubing. What is the total time to infuse?
    a. 25 min
    b. 025 h
    c. 4 h
    d. 4 min

16. Ordered: 500 mL ½ NSS at 75 mL/h. The infusion started at 1615, or 4:15 p.m. When will the infusion be completed?
    a. 11:25 p.m.
    b. 2125
    c. 11:45 p.m.
    d. 12:15 p.m.

17. Ordered: 1500 mL IV ⅓ NS q8h (10 gtt/mL tubing). What is the flow rate?
    a. 187.5 mL/h
    b. 31 gtt/min
    c. 31 mL/h
    d. 188 gtt/min

18. Ordered: 1000 mL RL over 8 h (15 gtt/mL tubing). After 2 h, 125 mL has infused. What is the adjusted flow rate in drops per minute?
    a. 36 mL/h
    b. 125 mL/h
    c. 36 gtt/min
    d. 31 gtt/min

19. Ordered: RL at 25 mL/h over 12 h. What is the volume to be administered?
    a. 2.5 mL
    b. 300 mL
    c. 400 mL
    d. 300 gtt/min

20. Ordered: 1000 mL at 125 mL/h, starting at 1 p.m. When will this infusion be completed?
    a. 9 a.m.
    b. 10 p.m.
    c. 9 p.m.
    d. 8 p.m.

21. Which of the following can be a calibration factor of IV tubing?
    a. 15 mL
    b. 15 mL/h
    c. 15 gtt/min
    d. 15 gtt/mL

What Should You Do? (Critical Thinking/Application Questions)

1. You are preparing an intermittent medication and you are not certain that your calculations are correct. What should you do?

_____

_____

_____

Get Connected

Visit the McGraw-Hill Higher Education website for *Intravenous Therapy for Health Care Personnel* at **www.mhhe.com/healthcareskills** to complete the following activities.

1. Search the Internet for additional examples of IV dosages and rate calculations. Remember, accuracy is mandatory and practice makes perfect. Use search terms such as *IV dosage calculations, IV infusion practice, and IV therapy math.* Many websites provide additional practice problems. Once you find a site, complete the problems and check your results. If requested, turn in your problems to your instructor.

Using the Student CD

Now that you have completed the material in Chapter 8, return to the student CD and complete any chapter activities you have not yet done. Practice your terminology with the Key Term Concentration game. Review the chapter material with the Spin the Wheel game. Take the final chapter test, complete the troubleshooting question, and e-mail or print your results to document your proficiency for this chapter.

Intravenous Fluid Abbreviations and Concentrations

D5W	5% dextrose in water
D10W	10% dextrose in water
NS, NSS	Normal saline (0.9% NaCl)
D5 NS	5% dextrose in normal saline
Ringer's	Ringer's solution
LR or RL	Lactated Ringer's or Ringer's lactate
D5 LR	5% dextrose in lactated Ringer's
½ NS, ½ NSS	Half normal saline solution (0.45% NaCl)
⅓ NS, ⅓ NSS	One-third normal saline solution (0.33% NaCl)
¼ NS, ¼ NSS	One-fourth normal saline solution (0.225% NaCl)

Solution	Category	Uses/Advantages	Disadvantages
Sodium Chloride (NaCl) Solutions			
0.225% NaCl (¼ NS)	Hypotonic	• ECF replacement when chloride loss is greater than or equal to sodium loss • Treatment for sodium depletion • Only solution that can be used with blood products	• Possible hypernatremia • Possible depletion of other electrolytes (such as potassium) • Possible circulatory overload due to expansion of the ECF compartment
0.45% NaCl (½ NS)	Hypotonic		
0.9% NaCl (NS)	Isotonic		
3% and 5% NaCl	Hypertonic		

(Continued)

Dextrose (D) Solutions

5% dextrose in water (D5W)	Isotonic	• Calories in the form of carbohydrates	• Blood vessel irritation, especially in higher concentrations
10% dextrose in water (D10W)	Hypertonic	• Free water • Treatment for hyperkalemia and dehydration	• Dehydration caused by rapid infusion of hypertonic solutions • Possible hyperinsulinemia
20% to 70% dextrose in water	Hypertonic	• Vehicle for medication administration	• Incompatibility with blood products and some medications

Solutions with a Combination of Sodium Chloride (NaCl) and Dextrose (D)

5% dextrose and .225% NaCl (D5 ½ NS)	Isotonic	• Temporary treatment of hypovolemic shock • Replacement of nutrients and electrolytes	• Possible hypernatremia, acidosis, and circulatory overload • Necessity of careful administration in patients with cardiac, renal, or liver disease
5% dextrose and .45% NaCl (D5 ½ NS)	Hypertonic	• Hydration of patients to assess kidney function	
5% dextrose and .9% NaCl (D5 NS)	Hypertonic	• Treatment of dehydration; promotion of diuresis	

Electrolyte Solutions

Ringer's solution	Isotonic	• Treatment of dehydration; restoration of fluid balance presurgery and postsurgery • Toleration by patients with liver disease • Short-term blood replacement • Similarity to normal saline, with the addition of potassium and calcium	• Lack of calories • Exacerbation of sodium retention, congestive heart failure, and renal insufficiency • Contraindication in renal failure
Lactated Ringer's or Ringer's lactate	Isotonic	• Treatment of all forms of dehydration, fluid losses from burns, mild metabolic acidosis, and salicylate (aspirin) overdose • Similarity to body's extracellular electrolyte content • Precursor of bicarbonate	• Possible hypernatremia • Contraindicated in patients with liver disease, hypovolemia, profound shock, or cardiac failure

Incompatible Intravenous Medications and Solutions

Medications placed in parenteral solutions may be incompatible with other medications and the IV solutions in which they are placed. Many incompatibilities can be detected in the tubing or syringe when medications are mixed. However, not all incompatibilities are evidenced by a visible change in a solution. The drug or drugs may become inactive without precipitating or changing color. Before adding a medication to a solution, hanging an IV piggyback, or mixing two medications, check their compatibility using a solution compatibility chart, medication reference book, or package insert or check with a pharmacist. The following is a list of some common incompatibilities:

Ampicillin in 5% dextrose in water
Cefotaxime sodium mixed with sodium bicarbonate
Diazepam mixed with potassium chloride
Dopamine hydrochloride mixed with sodium bicarbonate
Penicillin mixed with heparin
Penicillin mixed with vitamin B complex
Sodium bicarbonate in lactated Ringer's
Tetracycline hydrochloride mixed with calcium chloride
Blood given with anything *other* than normal saline

Common Intravenous Medications

acetazolamide
acyclovir
adenosine
alteplase
    recombinant
amikacin sulfate
aminocaproic acid
aminophylline
ammonium chloride
amphotericin
ampicillins
amprenavir
amrinone lactate
antithymocyte
    globulin
ascorbic acid
atropine sulfate
aztreonam
bretylium tosylate
bumetanide
buprenorphine
    hydrochloride
calcium salts
cefazolin sodium
cefepime
    hydrochloride
cefoperazone
    sodium
cefotaxime sodium
cefotetan disodium
cefoxitin sodium
ceftazidime
ceftizoxime sodium

ceftriaxone sodium
cefuroxime
chloramphenicol
chlordiazepoxide
    hydrochloride
chlorothiazide
cimetidine
ciprofloxacin
    hydrochloride
clindamycin
dexamethasone
dextran low
    molecular weight
diazepam
diazoxide
digoxin
dimenhydrinate
dobutamine
    hydrochloride
dopamine
    hydrochloride
doxycycline
epinephrine
epirubicin
    hydrochloride
esmolol
    hydrochloride
ethacrynic acid
famiotidine
fat emulsion
    intravenous
fentayl
fluconazole
folic acid

foscarnet sodium
furosemide
gatifloxacin
gentamicin sulfate
glucagon
heparin
hetastarch
hydralazine
    hydrochloride
hydromorphone
    hydrochloride
ibutilide fumaarate
insulin
interferon alfa n1
    lymphoblastoid
isoproterenol
kanamycin sulfate
labetalol
    hydrochloride
lidocaine
    hydrochloride
magnesium sulfate
mannitol
meperidine
    hydrochloride
meropenem
methyldopa
metoclopramide
metoprolol
metronidazole
morphine sulfate
multivitamin
    nafcillin sodium

naloxone
    hydrochloride
nitroglycerin
norepinephrine
ofloxacin
ondasetron
    hydrochloride
oxacillin sodium
oxytocin
pancuronium
pantoprazole
papaverine
penicillin G
    benzathine
pentamidine
    isethionate
pentobarbital
    sodium
perindopril
    erbumine
perphenazine
phenytoin
piperacillin sodium
potassium salts
procainamide
    hydrochloride
prochlorperazine
propranolol
    hydrochloride
protamine sulfate
pyridoxine
    hydrochloride
quinidine
ranitidine

ritodrine
  hydrochloride
sodium acetate
sodium bicarbonate
sodium chloride
streptokinase

succinyilcholine
theophylline
thiamine
thiopental
ticarcillin disodium
tobramycin sulfate

torsemide
trace metals
tranexamic acid
urokinase
vancomycin
  hydrochloride

verapamil
  hydrochloride
warfarin
zaleplon
zidovudine

Conversions, Abbreviations, and Formulas for Intravenous Calculations

Conversions and Measures

Metric Fluid Conversions
1 liter (L) = 1000 milliliters (mL)
1 milliliter (mL) = 0.001 liter (L)
1 milliliter (mL) = 1 cubic centimeter

Measures for Volume Approximations

Metric	Household	Apothecary
0.06 mL (*droppers vary*)	1 drop (gt)	1 drop (gt)
1 mL (*droppers vary*)	15 drops (gtt)	15 drops (gtt)
5 mL	1 tsp	1 dr (exact volume 3.7 mL)
15 mL	1 tbsp	3 or 4 dr
30 mL	2 tbsp or 1 oz	1 oz
240 mL	8 oz or 1 c	8 oz
480 mL	2 c = 1 pt	16 oz
960 mL (exact volume is 1000 mL)	1 qt or 2 pt or 4 c	32 oz

Abbreviations
gt = drop
gtt = drops
mL = milliliters (equivalent to cubic centimeter, or cc; however, cc abbreviations should not be used)
min = minutes

h = hour

gtt/min = drops per minute

mL/h = milliliters per hour

F = flow rate in milliliters per hour (mL/h)

V = volume

T = time

f = flow rate in drops per minute (gtt/min)

C = calibration factor of the tubing in drops per milliliter (gtt/mL)

D = desired dose (the amount of drug to be given at a single time)

Q = dosage unit (the unit by which the drug will be measured when administered)

H = the dose on hand (the amount of drug contained in each dosage unit)

A = amount to administer (the volume of liquid that contains the desired dose)

Calculations

Formula for calculating the flow rate in milliliters per hour (mL/h)

$$F = \frac{V}{T}$$

Formula for calculating the flow rate in drops per minute (gtt/min)

$$f = \frac{F \times C}{60 \text{ min/hr}}$$

Adjusting the flow rate

- Recalculate the infusion using the volume (V) remaining in the IV, the time (T) remaining in the order, and the calibration factor (C) of the tubing.
- Check the guidelines at your facility before adjusting the flow rate.

Formula for calculating the infusion time in hours (T)

$$T = \frac{V}{F}$$

Formula for calculating the infusion volume in milliliters (V)

$$V = T \times F$$

Formula for calculating the amount to administer (A)

$$A = \frac{D \times Q}{H}$$

Answer Key

Chapter One

Checkpoint Questions 1-1

1. An IV is used to infuse fluids, blood, blood products, and medications to patients who cannot take them by mouth.
2. Patients are given an IV when they cannot take foods, fluids, or medications by mouth; IVs are also used during emergency and critical-care situations.

Checkpoint Questions 1-2

1. IV therapy is regulated by OSHA, JCAHO, CDC, NIOSH, and HIPAA.
2. In order to reduce the number of needle-stick injuries, NIOSH has recommended and OSHA has implemented a regulation stating that safety devices must be used and that fines can be imposed if appropriate devices are not used.
3. OSHA has established universal and standard precautions to prevent infection during IV therapy.

Troubleshooting Determining Your Role

You would check the state law, your scope of practice, and the facility's policy before you remove the IV.

Checkpoint Questions 1-3

1. State that you are willing to learn the procedure if it is allowed by the state, the scope of practice, and the facility where you are working; however, currently you are not trained and would not feel comfortable doing the procedure without training.
2. Initiation of an IV and flushing an IV are considered invasive procedures.

3. Noninvasive IV therapy procedures include preparing IV equipment for placement, monitoring and maintaining an IV, and documenting IV therapy.

Checkpoint Questions 1-4

1. Four reasons for IV therapy are (1) to replace and maintain fluid and electrolyte balance; (2) to administer medications, including chemotherapeutic agents, intravenous anesthetics, and diagnostic reagents; (3) to transfuse blood and blood products; and (4) to deliver nutrients and nutritional supplements.
2. Cells move fluids and solutes by way of diffusion, active transport, osmosis, capillary filtration, and capillary reabsorption.
3. Fluid level in the body is regulated by thirst, urination, respiration, and hormones and in the cardiovascular system through fluid volume and pressure sensors.

Checkpoint Questions 1-5

1. The two types of IV therapy are peripheral and central.
2. Most patients receiving IV chemotherapy on an outpatient basis have an implantable port.

Chapter Review

Matching

1. f	5. c	9. e
2. b	6. a	10. j
3. i	7. g	
4. d	8. h	

True/False

11. True.

12. True.
13. False. Central lines or PICCs are best for long-term therapy because these catheters are inserted into larger veins and the solution is delivered into the central circulation. Peripheral IV catheters are inserted in smaller veins, which can infiltrate easily.
14. True.
15. False. Laws vary from state to state. The medical assistant must check state law prior to performing tasks associated with IV therapy.

Multiple Choice

16. b	**20.** b	**24.** b
17. c	**21.** a	**25.** d
18. c	**22.** d	
19. d	**23.** c	

Critical Thinking

1. The patient should be told about the IV and the reason it has been ordered. If providing this information is within your scope of practice, explain the procedure carefully and allow the patient to ask questions. If necessary, ask your supervisor to explain the procedure to the patient. In either case, the patient should receive a thorough explanation and should verbally agree to the IV before it is initiated.
2. HIPAA requires that you keep patient information confidential. You should not answer the questions unless the caller is properly identified and the patient has given written or, in some cases, verbal permission for the caller to be told information about her health care.

Get Connected

1. Review the legislation and scope of practice for the state in which you are located.
2. Using this web link http://www.jcaho.org/accredited+organizations/patient+safety/npsg.htm, select the location and field in which you will most likely be employed, such as ambulatory care or a hospital.

Chapter Two

Checkpoint Question 2-1

1. Poor safety and infection control measures during IV therapy can lead to financial expense, to the spread of infection, and to emotional distress from exposure to and treatment of infectious disease.

Checkpoint Questions 2-2

1. The Needlestick Safety and Prevention Act mandated changes that would reduce the number of needlestick injuries.
2. Adhere to the following precautions to prevent needlestick injuries: avoid the use of needles when possible, correctly use safe alternatives, do not recap needles, dispose of needles correctly, report hazards and needlestick injuries promptly, attend training, and follow established policies and procedures.

Checkpoint Questions 2-3

1. Safe-needle devices decrease the risk of needlestick injury and exposure to blood-borne pathogens.
2. When activating a safe-needle device, keep your hands behind the exposed needle, and make sure the safety feature is engaged.

Checkpoint Question 2-4

1. You must know if the LAD is a capped or capless device. If it is a capped device, you will need a new sterile cap to cover the port upon completion of the infusion. If it is a capless port, you will simply need to clean the top of the port with an alcohol prep pad prior to connecting the secondary set.

Checkpoint Questions 2-5

1. The chain of infection is the set of links needed for an infection to occur. If any one of the links is broken or blocked, an infection will not occur.
2. Standard Precautions are recommended for routine care of uninfected patients. Standard Precautions include hand hygiene and the wearing of gloves whenever you might come in contact with blood or body fluids.
3. You must wear an N95 or HEPA filter mask when entering the room of a patient who is under airborne precautions; you must also follow Standard Precautions while performing any care on this patient.

Troubleshooting Using Proper Hand Hygiene

If your hands are visibly soiled with blood or other contaminates, you should use soap and water. If your hands have no visible contamination, you can use the alcohol-based hand rub.

Checkpoint Questions 2-6

1. Gloves act as a protective barrier to prevent the contamination of the hands and to decrease the possibility of exposure to blood-borne pathogens.
2. A patient with tuberculosis is placed under airborne isolation precautions, and you should wear an N95 respirator or HEPA filter mask when entering the room.

Chapter Review

Matching

1. g	5. i	9. d
2. e	6. j	10. h
3. f	7. c	
4. a	8. b	

True/False

11. True.
12. False. Health care workers should avoid the use of needles when possible, correctly use safer alternatives, avoid recapping needles, dispose of needles promptly and appropriately, report hazards or injuries promptly, attend training, and follow policies and procedures related to infection control and use of needles.
13. True.
14. False. Standard Precautions are used with every patient during routine care. Isolation precautions are used with patients who have specific infections.
15. True.

Multiple Choice

16. d	20. b	24. d
17. a	21. d	25. c
18. b	22. c	
19. c	23. c	

Critical Thinking

1. You must report the incident to the supervisor. First, the needle left in the bed is a hazard that must be reported, and second, your coworker needs to be evaluated for possible exposure to blood-borne pathogens and to receive treatment if needed.
2. You should remove your gloves, explain to Mr. Johnson that you will assist him as soon as you wash your hands, then wash your hands and put on fresh gloves.

Get Connected

1. Your summary should include the CDC definition for an engineered sharps injury prevention device: a physical attribute built into any type of needle device or into a non-needle sharp that effectively reduces the risk of an exposure incident. These engineering modifications generally use one of the following strategies:
   - Elimination of the need for a needle (substitution)
   - Permanent isolation of the needle so that it never poses a hazard
   - A means to isolate or encase the needle after use
2. Your summary should describe any three of the devices listed on the NAPPSI website at www.nappsi.org/safety.shtml#ivInsertion.

Chapter Three

Checkpoint Question 3-1

1. A health care professional's most important function in IV therapy is to continuously monitor the patient and the infusion to ensure that the physician's orders are being carried out.

Checkpoint Question 3-2

1. The most common peripheral IV access device is the over-the-needle catheter. It has a safe-needle device, and it leaves only a hollow tube in place after insertion.

Checkpoint Questions 3-3

1. When choosing the appropriate venous access device, consider the following factors: the type of fluids to be administered; whether the patient will also receive IV medication; whether the patient will possibly need blood or blood products; the length of time that the patient is expected to be receiving IV fluids; whether the infusion will be continuous or intermittent; the location, size, and condition of the patient's veins; the age, level of activity, and consciousness of the patient.
2. The 18-gauge needle is larger and is more common; however, you should always select the shortest and smallest cannula that is sufficient to deliver the prescribed fluids, blood products, or medication.

Checkpoint Questions 3-4

1. Macrodrip tubing allows larger drops (10 to 15 drops/mL) to form and fall into the drip chamber; it is used for infusions of 80 mL/hour or more and is always used for operating room infusions. Microdrip tubing allows smaller drops (60 drops/mL) to enter the drip chamber; it is used for infusions of less than 80mL/hour and is often used for KVO infusions. Microdrip tubing is especially useful for pediatric and critical-care IVs, when very small volumes are used and accuracy is extremely important. Accidental increases in volume can be fatal in these situations.

2. Secondary administration sets are used for intermittent medications or fluids. They are piggybacked into the primary administration set.

Checkpoint Question 3-5

1. You may add a sticky label to the plastic IV fluid bag, or you may write on an already affixed label. Never mark directly on the fluid bag itself.

Troubleshooting PCA Pump Instruction

This patient has clearly not been taught how to use the PCA pump. If it is within your scope of practice, you should immediately give her the handheld button and explain that it is used for self-medication. Additionally, she should receive complete instructions about using the PCA pump, and a pain assessment should be done.

Checkpoint Questions 3-6

1. A gravity drip is used for manual infusion of IV fluids; the IV bag is hung 36 inches above the level of the patient and a clamp is used to regulate the flow rate.

2. Infusion pumps force the IV solution through the tubing. The pump applies pressure sufficient to deliver a set volume of liquid every minute into the patient's vein; the desired flow rate can be set either in mL/hour or by dosage. A sensor on the infusion pump sounds an alarm if the flow rate cannot be maintained or if the bag is empty.

3. Although both syringe pumps and PCA pumps have a syringe as part of the apparatus, the two devices serve different purposes: the syringe pump is used by the health care professional to administer medication at a precisely controlled rate whereas the PCA pump is used by the patient to self-administer pain medication.

Chapter Review

Multiple Choice

1. c	3. c	5. b
2. d	4. b	

Fill-in-the-Blank

6. pump
7. faster
8. blood pressure
9. wing-tipped (butterfly) or steel needle
10. larger or wider

Matching

11. b	15. c	19. h
12. e	16. j	20. a
13. f	17. d	
14. i	18. g	

Identification

21. c	25. f	29. g
22. e	26. a	30. b
23. d	27. h	
24. i	28. j	

True/False

31. True.
32. True.
33. True.
34. False. Implantable ports have a lower incidence of infection because the skin is a natural barrier against infection.
35. True.

Critical Thinking

1. Your first action is to check the flow rate, even if an electronic infusion pump is being used. Like any electronic device, it can malfunction. Assessing the flow rate manually can tell you the exact rate of the infusion. Because of the many variables that can affect the flow rate of individual patients, IV infusion pumps are more accurate than are IVs with a gravity drip, but only if they are calibrated and working correctly.

Get Connected

1. Using this website, http://www.lite.org, you can access information about the League of Intravenous Therapy Education.
2. Identify the journal you have selected, and print out the e-copy of your journal article for use in class review and discussion. One good source for journals is the Nursing Center website at http://www.nursingcenter.com, which offers journal articles as well as information on continuing education opportunities.

Chapter Four

Checkpoint Questions 4-1

1. In a dehydrated patient, the serum osmolarity is higher than normal.
2. In a patient with a fluid overload, the serum osmolarity is lower than normal.
3. NS stands for normal saline; LR stands for lactated Ringer's; D stands for dextrose.

Checkpoint Questions 4-2

1. The three categories of IV fluids based on osmolarity are isotonic, hypertonic, and hypotonic. Isotonic fluids have the same concentration, or osmolarity, that serum does. Hypertonic fluids are more concentrated and, therefore, have a higher osmolarity than serum does. Hypotonic fluids are less concentrated and have a lower osmolarity than serum does.
2. The blood donor and the recipient must be ABO- and Rh-compatible to prevent hemolytic transfusion reactions.

Troubleshooting Patients Receiving Heparin

You should watch for bleeding gums, nosebleeds, increased bruising, or black tarry stools. Use a sponge swab or soft toothbrush to provide mouth care. Use an electric razor or avoid shaving a male patient until his PR/INR stabilizes. If the patient is alert and oriented, instruct the patient about precautions to take and signs and symptoms to report.

Troubleshooting Patients Receiving Insulin

You should report the patient's symptoms to the health care professional in charge. You should also do a fingerstick blood glucose check immediately to find out the patient's blood sugar level. She is showing signs of hypoglycemia.

Checkpoint Questions 4-3

1. Parenteral nutrition is the IV infusion of nutrients, including amino acids, dextrose, fat, electrolytes, vitamins, and trace elements.
2. Heparin keeps clots from getting bigger and prevents new clots from forming.
3. When potassium is added to an IV solution, the bag should be agitated because potassium can be irritating to the vein; also, the patient must be monitored for signs of phlebitis or infiltration. Calcium must not be administered with bicarbonate solutions because precipitate may form; also, calcium can cause severe tissue damage if infiltration occurs.

Checkpoint Question 4-4

1. Some factors that affect compatibility are the order in which drugs are mixed, drug concentrations, length of time that drugs are in contact with other drugs or solutions, temperature, exposure to light, and pH.

Checkpoint Questions 4-5

1. The advantages to administering medications by IV: medications can reach the bloodstream quickly in emergencies; medications can be stopped quickly; administration is less painful than intramuscular or subcutaneous administrations are; medications can be administered to patients who cannot take medications orally. The disadvantages: IV administration can cause incompatibility issues; errors can occur when medications are reconstituted; patients can develop phlebitis or extravasation; too rapid an infusion can lead to speed shock.
2. The seven rights of medication administration are right medication, right patient, right time, right route, right method (technique), right dose, and right documentation.

Chapter Review

Matching

1. d		5. j		9. c	
2. f		6. b		10. e	
3. h		7. i			
4. a		8. g			

True/False

11. True.

12. False. Plasma expanders are used to increase a patient's circulating volume by expanding the intravascular space.
13. True.
14. True.
15. False. Incompatibility that results in a physical or chemical change in the solution may cause the loss of therapeutic effects of a medication.

Multiple Choice

16. c	20. b	24. c
17. a	21. c	25. a
18. d	22. d	
19. d	23. b	

Critical Thinking

1. First, you should not hang the IV antibiotic. Second, you should check the patient's medical record for a list of allergies to see if the medication is on it. Third, regardless of whether the medication is noted on the patient's list of allergies, you should report the incident to your supervisor. If the patient's record does not list any allergies but the patient states that he has an allergy, the patient's record must be corrected. If the antibiotic is on the patient's list of allergies, the physician must be contacted to change the medication.

2. You must change the IV bag immediately. To prevent incompatibilities caused by the length of time that drugs are in contact with other drugs or solutions, IV bags are changed every 24 hours regardless of how much solution remains in the bag.

Get Connected

1. Two suggested websites at which you may find information are the U.S. Department of Veterans Affairs at www.va.gov and the Institute for Safe Medication Practices at www.ismp.org. Your written policy should include the names of several medications considered to be high-alert and should provide detailed instructions on how these medications are to be handled.

Chapter Five

Checkpoint Questions 5-1

1. The basic preparatory steps before initiating an IV are verifying the physician's orders, gathering the equipment, introducing yourself to the patient, identifying the patient, providing for patient privacy, washing your hands, and putting on gloves.

2. You must adhere to Standard Precautions because when you initiate an IV infusion, the patient's skin and vein will be punctured. You must protect yourself from contact with the patient's blood by wearing gloves and, if the situation warrants it, a gown, mask, or goggles. You must follow strict aseptic technique because contamination of fluids, equipment, or supplies could introduce bacteria into the patient's bloodstream.

Troubleshooting Reading a Physician's Order

You are infusing normal sterile saline, or normal saline. The rate of the fluid is 125 mL per hour, and the fluid bag contains 1000 mL.

Checkpoint Questions 5-2

1. The physician's order should specify the type of fluid, the amount of fluid, and the rate of infusion.

2. Explain the procedure to the patient, including the rationale, or why; what the patient can do to help the procedure run smoothly; what the patient should avoid doing; and roughly how long the IV infusion will be in progress. Recognize the patient's fears, and allow the patient to express them.

3. Allow the patient to use the bathroom, help the patient change into an IV gown if available, prepare the site by clipping body hair if necessary, and use an anesthetic if directed to do so (follow facility guidelines and manufacturer's directions).

Checkpoint Questions 5-3

1. Match the MAR or IV administration sheet against the patient's name and medical record that appear on the identification band that the patient is wearing. Always use two identifiers.

2. Prior to initiating IV therapy, check the following items: physician's orders; patient's medical history, especially allergies and conditions that might affect selection of infusion site or equipment, for example, a mastectomy or paralysis; whether the patient be receiving IV medication or just fluids; whether an infusion pump will be used.

3. When preparing IV medications for more than one patient, prepare each patient's medication separately. First, check the physician's order for any changes or additions. Second, prepare only that patient's dose in the medication room, and take only one medication at a time to the patient's room. Third, match the infusion bag label against the MAR or IV administration sheet as well as against the patient's identification band. Only after you have successfully attached one patient's medication do you turn to the next patient.

Checkpoint Questions 5-4

1. The preferred order of IV sites in the hand and arm are the dorsal surface of the hand (dorsal digital or dorsal metacarpal), superficial radial and ulnar veins on the forearm (median antebrachial), cephalic vein on the radial border of the forearm, then the basilica vein on the ulnar portion of the forearm.
2. An IV inserted into a patient's antecubital fossa requires the patient to keep that arm straight for the fluid to flow properly. The arm board that is typically used for this purpose is uncomfortable for the patient.

Checkpoint Questions 5-5

1. The supplies that you will need before initiating an IV are an IV cannula of the appropriate size, a fluid administration set, the prescribed fluid, the MAR and/or IV flow sheet, a vital signs graphic sheet or flow chart, and cannulation and site supplies.
2. Some ways that you can prevent the spread of infection are to wash your hands or use an alcohol hand cleanser before you start, to not contaminate the puncture spike or the tip of the tubing when you purge the line.

Checkpoint Questions 5-6

1. To keep the vein from rolling during IV insertion, apply traction on the skin below the site with your nondominant hand.
2. *Flash* refers to the blood that is seen when the IV cannula enters the vein; the blood appears in the flash chamber of the cannula. This blood is also called *flashback*.

Checkpoint Questions 5-7

1. When giving IV therapy to a geriatric patient, avoid using the back of the hand, apply hand pressure instead of a tourniquet (in some cases), and monitor fluid intake carefully.
2. Techniques to facilitate IV therapy on an obese patient are to apply warm compresses for vasodilation, to depress the extra tissue at the site and mark the spot or cannula quickly, to use the vein on the thumb side of the wrist, and to use multiple tourniquets distally from the most proximal joint toward the site.

Chapter Review

Multiple Choice

1. d	4. b	7. d
2. c	5. c	8. b
3. b	6. c	9. b

Number the Steps

10.

13 release the tourniquet
16 tape the IV tubing to the skin
 6 select the insertion site
 8 put on gloves
 2 select the equipment
10 insert the cannulation device
 4 prepare the patient
 5 dilate and palpate the vein
 3 prepare the solution set
 1 review the order for IV access
12 withdraw the needle
17 document the procedure
 7 select the cannulation device
14 connect the fluid-filled tubing to the hub
11 advance the cannulation device
15 apply a clear sterile dressing
 9 prepare the site

Matching

11. i	15. c	19. b
12. f	16. j	20. g
13. d	17. e	
14. h	18. a	

True/False

21. False. A large-diameter needle, such as 18 gauge, should be used for blood transfusions.

22. True.
23. True.
24. False. Arteries are never used for intravenous therapy.
25. False. Veins carry blood toward the heart.

Critical Thinking

1. You must attempt to obtain a medical history from the patient or a family member if available; you could also call the number on the medic alert tag to obtain any information that is on file. You should inform the ER physician that the patient has a history of diabetes, and ask the physician if you should proceed with the IV infusion.
2. First, you will check the infusion pump to be sure it is set properly. Second, you will remove the gauze and replace it with a transparent dressing so the site can be observed more easily. Third, you will remove and replace any tape strips that are constrictive, taking care not to disturb the cannula. Fourth, you will check for a blood return when the fluid container is lowered. If blood return is present, you will continue to observe the site; if not, you will discontinue the IV and replace it at a new site.

Get Connected

1. The link for the MedlinePlus dictionary is http://www.nlm.nih.gov/medlineplus/mplusdictionary.html.

Chapter Six

Checkpoint Questions 6-1

1. When you take over the care of a patient with an IV, you need to know when the IV was started, whether it is infusing on schedule, and the condition of the IV site.
2. The patient record and labels on the IV bag and insertion site will provide you with the information you need to care for a patient with an IV.

Checkpoint Questions 6-2

1. Label the IV site with the date and time of the dressing change, the date and time that the IV was started, the gauge and length of the catheter, and your initials.

2. The time strip on an IV solution allows the health care worker to quickly monitor the infusion rate.

Troubleshooting Rising Cost vs Patient Care

You should prepare, properly label, and hang a new bag and tubing. IV fluids should be changed every 24 hours and tubing every 72 hours. Because the current bag and tubing were not labeled, it is not possible to know when it was hung. Not changing it increases the patient's risk for developing complications such as phlebitis. Although all health care personnel should be aware of reducing health care costs, the care of the patient should never be compromised.

Checkpoint Questions 6-3

1. The two types of dressings used on IV sites are the transparent semipermeable membrane dressing and the sterile gauze and tape dressing.
2. Change an IV dressing every 48 hours if made of gauze, every 72 hours if made of a semipermeable membrane, and whenever you find that the dressing has become loose or soiled.

Checkpoint Questions 6-4

1. The patient's IV can infiltrate, or the patient can develop phlebitis. Other complications of IV therapy include fluid overload, hypersensitivity reaction, infection, and air embolus.
2. Infiltration is the seepage of IV solution into the tissues around the IV catheter, causing swelling, discomfort, tightness, cool skin, and blanching. Phlebitis is an inflammation of the vein due to irritation, and it causes redness, tenderness, puffiness, warmth, and possible fever. Both conditions result in the slowing or stopping of the IV flow rate. Treatments for both include early detection, removal of the IV catheter, and warm or cold compresses.

Checkpoint Questions 6-5

1. If you encounter a problem with an IV flow rate, troubleshoot to see why the IV is not infusing at the correct rate, make appropriate corrections, and recalculate and reset the rate.
2. IV infusion rates can be affected by patient-related factors, equipment-related factors, or vein-related factors.

Chapter Review

Matching

1. c   **3.** e   **5.** a
2. f   **4.** b   **6.** d

True/False

7. True.

8. False. Phlebitis is the inflammation of the inner lining of a vein due to mechanical or chemical causes. Extravasation is the leakage of vesicant fluids into tissues surrounding an IV site.

9. False. Checking for blood return is not a reliable method for determining if an IV has infiltrated. You should apply gentle pressure over the vein below the catheter tip. If the IV continues to drip, it is probably infiltrated.

10. True.

11. True.

Multiple Choice

12. b   **16.** a   **20.** c
13. c   **17.** c   **21.** d
14. d   **18.** c
15. c   **19.** b

Critical Thinking

1. This patient has Grade 1 phlebitis. You should remove his IV and place warm compresses at the site if these actions are within your scope of practice. You would document your actions as follows: "IV site red. Patient complaint of pain at site. IV removed and warm compresses applied." Always include your initials or full name, the date, and the time with the documentation.

2. You should take the following actions to check your patient's IV infusion pump: systematically assess the infusion beginning with the pump; check all the settings; check the drip chamber and the clamps. All clamps should be open, and fluid should be dripping into the chamber. Examine the length of the tubing for the presence of air or kinks. Also, be sure that the tubing is not caught on any furniture or equipment. Assess the insertion site. Look at the tape to be sure it is not too tight; if it is constricting the skin or tissue, it could also be constricting the flow. Correct any problems with the tape. Check the site for swelling, redness, or leaking fluid. Lower the fluid container to below the site to check for blood return. If you do not see any blood return or any other signs of infiltration, discontinue the IV and restart it in another location.

Get Connected

1. The IV Team link is http://www.ivteam.com. Your summary should explain how to prevent three complications of IV therapy.

Chapter Seven

Checkpoint Question 7-1

1. Care and procedures that are not documented are not considered done. Health care facilities, health care regulating agencies, and lawyers handling malpractice lawsuits will all be expecting accurate and thorough documentation. Incomplete or inaccurate documentation can cause problems for the health care employee.

Checkpoint Questions 7-2

1. Document IV therapy when it is initiated, during the course of treatment, and when it is discontinued.

2. In documenting your assessment, include the amount and type of IV fluids administered; other fluid intake and output; any signs or symptoms of fluid deficit or excess; any signs or symptoms of sodium and potassium deficit or excess. Also include your observation of the IV site; note any redness, signs of infection, swelling, or temperature change.

3. Ask the patient to rate the pain on a scale of 1 to 10 with 1 being the least amount of pain and 10 being the greatest amount of pain. If you are using an infusion pump you may want to disconnect the IV from the pump and determine if it will flow with gravity only. Document your findings then continue to observe the site for redness, swelling, and slowed infusion rate handling a problem with an IV.

Checkpoint Questions 7-3

1. Document the patient's pain on a scale of 1 to 10, and document the patient's temperature, including the route you used to take it.

2. If you cannot resolve a problem with an IV infusion, check with a colleague or your supervisor before discontinuing the IV; document the problem and the actions taken.

Checkpoint Questions 7-4

1. I&O record sheets are kept for patients who cannot maintain fluid balance due to illness and have to be put on IV infusions.
2. IV TBA is the amount of fluid left in the solution container at the time you total the patient's fluid balance record or at the end of your shift. IV absorbed is the total amount of fluid absorbed during your shift.

Checkpoint Questions 7-5

1. After discontinuing an IV, apply pressure to the insertion site for 2 to 3 minutes or until the bleeding stops.
2. Stabilize the catheter when you discontinue an IV because movement of the catheter can cause pain to the patient or can cause bleeding and injury to the vein.

Chapter Review

Multiple Choice

1. c	5. d	9. a
2. d	6. a	10. c
3. b	7. c	11. d
4. c	8. b	

Matching

12. c	14. a	16. b
13. e	15. d	

Fill-in-the-Blank

17. anticoagulants
18. fluid loss
19. JCAHO
20. catheter tip
21. output

True/False

22. False. The abbreviation "MS" should not be used because it can be confused for "magnesium sulfate." You should write out "morphine sulfate."
23. True.
24. True.
25. False. Patient education is always documented as part of IV therapy. Some facilities provide a special place on the medical record for documenting patient education.
26. True.

Critical Thinking

1. Explain to your patient that steady pressure over the insertion site for 2 to 3 minutes usually stops any bleeding but that because this patient is on aspirin therapy, she may bleed for a longer period of time and she may be more susceptible to hematoma formation. Tell the patient that flexing her arm may increase the size of the wound in the vessel wall, resulting in additional bruising at the site.

Get Connected

1. The link for JCAHO is http://www.jcaho.org.

Chapter Eight

Checkpoint Question 8-1

1. For an IV infusion, you must be able to calculate the rate in milliliters per hour and/or drops per minute, the infusion time and volume, and the medication amount, time and volume.

Checkpoint Question 8-2

1. The flow rates for this order are 63 mL/h and 16 gtt/min.

Troubleshooting Recalculating a Flow Rate

You should recalculate the IV flow rate with the remaining amount of time (4 h) and volume left (450 mL). Do not try to catch up the IV fluid in the next hour; this would be outside the guidelines set by the facility. The new flow rate is 19 gtt/min.

Checkpoint Question 8-3

1. The original flow rate was 125 mL/h, or 31 gtt/min. The flow rate can be safely adjusted to 146 mL/h, or 36 gtt/min.

Checkpoint Questions 8-4

1. The total infusion time is 12 hours and 3 minutes.
2. The infusion will be completed at 0800, or 8 a.m. the next day.
3. The total volume administered is 800 mL.

Checkpoint Question 8-5

1. The amount to administer is 75 mL. The flow rate in milliliters per hour is 150 mL/h. The flow rate in drops per minute is 25 gtt/min.

Chapter Review

Matching

1. c	3. d	5. f
2. e	4. a	6. b

True/False

7. True.
8. False. IV flow rate adjustments are always based on the amount of time left for the infusion and the amount of fluid left in the bag.
9. False. Intermittent peripheral infusion devices are also known as saline or heparin locks and are used to administer fluids or medications on a schedule.
10. True.
11. True.

Multiple Choice

12.	b	16.	a	20.	c
13.	c	17.	b	21.	d
14.	d	18.	c		
15.	c	19.	b		

Critical Thinking

1. You should always double-check your calculation and/or ask for assistance. An error is not acceptable.

Get Connected

1. Some possible websites that you can use are http://chhs.gsu.edu/nursing/docs/CalculationQuizN3510.pdf, http://chhs.gsu.edu/nursing/docs/CalculationQuizN3510.pdf, www.cnhs.umb.edu/current/guides/same/SAMEPrep%202.1studyguidePDF.pdf

Competency Checklists

The following Competency Checklists can be used in the classroom or laboratory setting. In the classroom portion of training, you can review the procedures presented in the book in a step by step format. The competency checklists further divide each procedure in to pre-procedure, procedure, and post-procedure section for simplicity and ease of review. If you are learning the hands-on procedures for intravenous therapy the checklist format provides a place to mark proficiency and whether the task has been mastered. Critical steps include rationale or a reason why the step is so essential to mastering the task.

COMPETENCY CHECKLIST 5-1
Preparing for a Peripheral IV

Procedure Step	Rationale	Performed Yes	No	Mastered
Pre-Procedure				
1. Wash hands.	Maintains infection control.			
2. Compare type, amount, and rate of fluids with physician's order.	Maintains accuracy.			
3. Check pharmacy label for patient's identification, fluid type, additives, and expiration date.				
4. Select appropriate IV administration set.				
5. Select add-on filter, if indicated.				
6. Obtain appropriate venous access device and supplies.				
7. Remove outer wrapper from IV fluid bag.				
8. Inspect bag for tears or leaks visually and by applying gentle pressure to bag.				
9. Hold bag against dark and light backgrounds to examine for discoloration, cloudiness, or particulate matter.	Any evidence of change is an indication of contamination. If found, discard and replace with a new fluid container.			
Equipment Preparation for Manual Control				
10. Hang IV bag on IV pole.				
11. Close tubing roller clamp.				
12. Remove plastic protector from IV port.				
13. Squeeze drip chamber and insert tubing spike into bag port, holding the port securely to prevent contamination.	Squeezing the chamber during insertion prevents air from entering the bag.			
14. Release pressure on the drip chamber until chamber is half-full.				

15. Attach add-on terminal filter (if indicated).

16. Remove protective cap at end of tubing.

17. Open clamp on line to prime tubing and filter.

18. Hold tubing tip higher than tubing-dependent loop while priming.

Air rises and passes out as the tube is primed with fluid.

19. Invert and tap Y injection site as tubing primes.

20. Hold filter (if attached) point downward so proximal half of filter fills with fluid first, then invert to complete priming, tapping air out as filter primes.

Removes all air from line.

21. Close tubing clamp when primed.

Stops flow of solution.

22. Replace protective cap. (This will be attached to access device after IV cannulation is completed.)

Maintains asepsis.

Equipment Preparation When Using an Electronic Flow-Control Device

10. Spike IV fluid bag.

11. Close regulating clamp on set tubing before hanging bag.

12. Fill drip chamber to minimum one-third full.

This amount allows for sufficient air space in the drip chamber.

13. Prime tubing by opening regulating clamp slowly and allow tubing to fill with IV fluid. (If using cassette-type tubing, follow package instructions to correctly fill cassette portion of tubing.)

Allows for slight differences with each pump.

14. Follow manufacturer's instructions, and load administration set into device, taking care to fit tubing or cassette into appropriate receptor site.

Pump will not function if improperly loaded.

15. Close device door and latch.

16. Don gloves.

(Continued)

Procedure Step	Rationale	Performed Yes No	Mastered

Equipment Preparation When Using an Electronic Flow-Control Device (*continued*)

17. Establish venous access according to Procedure 5-2.

18. Connect administration set tubing to established infusion site.

19. Open regulating clamp on administration set. — Clamp must be open for pump to function.

20. Turn on device.

21. Set device parameters for operation, following manufacturer's instructions or machine set-up prompts. Parameters may include:
    a. Infusion (primary)
    b. Volume to be infused
    c. Rate (mL/hr)
    d. Pressure

22. Start device when parameters are set.

Post-Procedure

23. Observe that infusion is running properly. — Always check electronic equipment for proper functioning.

24. Remove gloves and wash hands. — Maintains infection control.

25. Document appropriately. — Provides communication with other members of the health care team.

Comments _____

_____

_____

_____

Signed:

Evaluator _____

Student _____

COMPETENCY CHECKLIST 5-2

Initiating a Peripheral IV

Procedure Step	Rationale	Performed Yes	No	Mastered
Pre-Procedure				
1. Explain procedure to patient.	Gains patient's cooperation and alleviates fears.			
2. Provide privacy.	Maintains confidentiality and meets HIPAA regulations.			
3. Hang fluid bag and primed administration set within easy reach.	Makes it available when you are ready to connect it.			
4. Position patient and adjust light.	Having the patient at the proper height and having adequate light helps prevent injury to yourself and helps you visualize the veins.			
5. Cut tape and place on clean table edge.	Tape is easier to prepare prior to donning gloves.			
6. Wash hands and don gloves.	Maintains infection control.			
7. Select appropriate venous access device.	Ensures use of the shortest, smallest device that gets the job done.			
Site Selection When Using a Tourniquet				

8. Select vein on patient's nondominant arm if possible.
  a. Inspect both arms, palpating and visualizing the course of veins.
  b. Select a superficial, easily palpated, and large enough vein.
  c. Check area for lesions or scars and select an area away from joints.
  d. Do not use antecubital fossa except as last resort.
  e. Do not use the same vein below an infiltration or site of phlebitis.
  f. Select shortest and smallest cannula sufficient for delivery.
  g. Select distal end of vein first.
  h. Select larger vein for blood transfusion or hypertonic fluid.
  i. Avoid vein in affected arm following mastectomy or other circulatory impairment.
  j. Use lower extremity *only* if necessary and allowed by your facility.
	Ensures a successful cannulation; prevents complications and prevents injury to patient.			

9. Apply tourniquet a few inches above the elbow to observe potential veins; then apply tourniquet 4 to 6 inches above selected site to distend vein. Secure tourniquet with loop to impede venous return but ensure arterial flow.	Properly distends vein without undue discomfort or injury.			

(Continued)

Procedure Step	Rationale	Performed Yes	No	Mastered

Site Selection When Using Blood Pressure Cuff instead of Tourniquet

8. Inflate blood pressure cuff just below diastolic reading.
   a. Tap vein lightly to distend.
   b. Ask patient to open and close fist.
   c. If palpating is difficult, apply warm, moist compress to area for 10 to 20 minutes.
   d. Position patient's arm dependent for few minutes to assist with distending vein.

   Rationale: Using a blood pressure cuff provides more even pressure to distend a difficult-to-visualize vein.

9. Check for presence of radial pulse.

   Rationale: Ensures that there is still arterial flow.

Using an Over-the-Needle Catheter to Initiate the IV

10. Prep site with antimicrobial swab.

    Rationale: Maintains infection control.

11. Let prep solution dry naturally.

    Rationale: Touching, wiping, or fanning the area to dry can negate the action of the solution.

12. Do not touch selected insertion site after prepping.

13. Hold catheter with bevel of needle up; insert needle/catheter unit at 45° angle into patient's skin.

14. Apply traction to stabilize patient's skin.

15. Re-visualize vein; reduce angle of cannula, pierce vein, and observe for backflow of blood into hub while continuing to apply traction.

16. Hold needle and gently advance plastic catheter hub over needle and up vein no more than half.

17. Stop and separate, but do not completely remove stylet from catheter.

18. Advance only the catheter until hub meets skin.

19. Release tourniquet. Leave stylet in catheter while taping catheter to skin.

20. Tape across body of hub without touching hub/catheter junction.

21. Place digital pressure over distal end of catheter and carefully remove stylet.

22. Maintain aseptic technique; connect catheter to IV tubing.

Using a Winged Needle to Initiate the IV

10. Select winged needle for adults, children, infants, and elderly clients who have small or fragile veins.

11. Affix end of IV infusion tubing to end of winged needle tubing. Remove sterile cover from needle to run fluid through needle; prime tubing, then clamp tube.

12. Apply tourniquet or blood pressure cuff to distend selected vein.

13. Prep the site.

14. Remove protective cap from winged needle; hold by its wings.

15. Anchor vein by placing thumb of nondominant hand below selected site and pulling skin taut. With bevel up, enter patient's skin at a 30° angle.

16. Follow course of vein until vein is entered, when lack of resistance is felt.

    Inserting needle through skin and into a small vein with one thrust may result in a hematoma.

17. Observe for flash of blood in needle tubing.

    Helps to ascertain that the vein has been entered.

18. Carefully advance needle up course of vein.

19. Release tourniquet.

    Allows for resumption of blood flow.

20. Affix IV tubing, open clamp, and observe drip chamber.

    Fluid should flow easily, and there should be no sudden swelling at the site.

21. Reduce flow rate to KVO until secured in place.

22. Securely tape wings.

    Prevents movement of device.

Comments _____

_____

_____

_____

Signed:

Evaluator _____

Student _____

COMPETENCY CHECKLIST 7-1

Discontinuing an IV

Procedure Step	Rationale	Performed Yes	No	Mastered
Pre-Procedure				
1. Gather equipment: 2×2 sterile gauze, tape, clean gloves.				
2. Wash hands and don gloves.	Maintains infection control and Standard Precautions.			
3. Explain procedure to patient.	Alleviates patient's concern and gains cooperation.			
Procedure				
4. Turn off infusion.	Prevents getting bed wet.			
5. Loosen dressing and tape.	Minimizes trauma to puncture site.			
6. Stabilize needle or catheter while removing dressing and tape.	Prevents unnecessary movements that could injure the vein.			
7. Hold sterile gauze over site and remove catheter carefully and smoothly, keeping it almost flush with skin. Do not put pressure on needle while it is still in vein.	Pressure on the needle point or catheter could cause injury to the vein.			
8. Immediately press a 2×2 sterile gauze over the site. Continue to apply firm pressure until bleeding stops.	Stops bleeding and lessens the risk of contact with blood.			
9. If the patient is on medication that prolongs bleeding time, maintain pressure for several minutes.	Patients taking aspirin or anticoagulants take a longer time to clot and are prone to bruising.			
10. Replace with a clean pad and tape in place.	Maintains infection control and patient comfort.			
11. Elevate patient's arm to reduce venous pressure and to facilitate clot formation. Do not bend patient's elbow.	Bending the elbow may cause a hematoma formation.			
12. Observe venipuncture site for redness, swelling, or hematoma.	Ensures early treatment of complications.			
13. Dispose of equipment and gloves properly.	Maintains infection control and safety.			

(Continued)

Post-Procedure

14. Wash your hands.	Maintains infection control.
15. Check site again in 15 minutes.	Ensures proper documentation and recognition of any impending complications.
16. Record volume infused on intake and output record.	Documents result of infusion.

Comments _____

_____

_____

_____

Signed:

Evaluator _____

Student _____

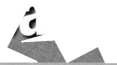

A

ABO system   Blood grouping system based on antigens present on red blood cells and antibodies in the serum; the most important system for determining donor/recipient compatibility.

Active transport   Transport of solutes from an area of lower concentration across a membrane to an area of higher concentration; requires energy.

Airborne transmission   The method by which pathogens from a reservoir are spread by air currents and inhaled by a susceptible host.

Aldosterone   Hormone secreted by the adrenal glands that affects fluid balance by causing the retention of sodium when the circulating fluid is low, when the sodium level is low, or when the potassium level is high.

Amount to administer (A)   The volume of liquid that contains the desired dose.

Anaphylaxis   Life-threatening allergic reaction to a medication or other foreign substance; symptoms include fainting, itching, hives, hypotension, and severe respiratory distress.

Anesthetic cream   A solid medication applied to the skin prior to venipuncture that reduces the sensation on the skin, thus reducing the pain of needle insertion. One brand of anesthetic cream is EMLA.

Antecubital   The area on the arm inside the elbow; the site commonly used for phlebotomy.

Anticoagulants   Medications such as heparin and warfarin that affect the ability of the blood to clot.

Antidiuretic hormone (ADH)   Hormone secreted from the pituitary gland that regulates the retention of water.

B

Blanching   The whitish color that appears when pressure is applied to an area of the patient's skin.

Blood components   Products separated from a unit of whole blood, such as platelets and red blood cells.

Blood-borne pathogen   Microorganisms that are present in blood and cause disease in humans.

Bronchospasm   Constriction of the air passages, causing difficulty breathing.

C

Calibration factor   The number of drops needed to deliver 1 mL of fluid through IV tubing; this number is based on the size or calibration of the tubing; also known as drop factor.

Cannula system   A venous access device in the form of a plastic tube, the lumen of which, during insertion, is usually occupied by a trocar (needle); once the tube is in place, the needle is removed and discarded.

Cannulation   The act of inserting a venous access device into a vein for intravenous therapy.

Capillary filtration   Type of fluid transport that forces fluid and solutes through the capillary wall pores from the intravascular fluid into the interstitial fluid.

Capillary reabsoprtion   Type of fluid transport that keep capillary filtration from removing an excess of intravascular fluid.

Centers for Disease Control and Prevention (CDC)   An agency of the U.S. government that protects the health and safety of individuals through prevention and control of infectious and chronic disease, injuries, workplace hazards, disabilities, and environmental health threats.

Central IV therapy   Infusions of fluids or medications directly into a larger vein such as the superior vena cava.

Central venous line   A small, flexible plastic tube, called a catheter, inserted into the large vein above the heart through which access to the bloodstream can be made; these catheters can be left in place for many weeks to months; also known as a central line.

Chain of infection   A group of six steps that must take place for an infection to occur: reservoir, infectious agent, portal of exit, mode of transmission, portal of entry, and susceptible host.

Compatibility   The ability for solutions or medications to be mixed and administered without an undesirable chemical or physical change occurring and without loss of therapeutic effect.

Contact transmission   The method by which pathogens are spread through either direct or indirect contact between the reservoir and a susceptible host.

D

Desired dose (*D*)   The amount of drug to be given at a single time.

Diffusion   A passive process that moves solutes from an area of higher concentration across a membrane to an area of lower concentration.

Dosage unit (*Q*)   The unit by which the drug will be measured when administered.

Dose on hand (*H*)   The amount of drug contained in each dosage unit.

Drop factor   The number of drops needed to deliver 1 mL of fluid through IV tubing; this number is based on the size or calibration of the tubing; also known as calibration factor.

Droplet transmission   Method by which pathogens are spread from the reservoir to the susceptible host through beads of moisture containing the pathogen, such as from a sneeze.

E

Ecchymosis   Bruise; black-and-blue discoloration of the skin due to blood leaking into the tissues from injured vessels.

Electrolytes   Substances that detach into electrically charged particles or ions that conduct electricity necessary for normal cell function.

Electronic flow control device   Any type of IV regulator that uses power to control or regulate the flow of IV fluids.

EMLA   Brand name of an anesthetic cream made by AstraZeneca that reduces the pain of needlestick procedures.

Erythema   Redness of the skin resulting from inflammation.

Extension tubing   Tubing added to the primary administration set to provide additional length or medications.

Extracellular fluid (ECF)   Fluids outside the cells.

Extravasation   The inadvertent infiltration of necrotizing or vesicant (blister-producing) solutions or medications into surrounding tissue.

F

Flash   The appearance of blood in the venous access device once successful cannulation has occurred.

G

gtt/min   Drops per minute; the flow rate value for manually controlled IV infusions.

H

Hematoma   A localized accumulation of partially clotted blood outside a blood vessel.

Hemolytic reaction   Blood transfusion reaction caused by a donor/recipient incompatibility.

Heparin flush   An injection of a diluted solution of the anticoagulant medication heparin that prevents clotting and keeps any IV access device open and flowing freely.

High-alert medication   Medication that can cause significant patient harm if used incorrectly.

Hypersensitivity reaction   Allergic reaction; response of the immune system to a medication, solution, or other substance. The reaction may range from a simple rash to anaphylaxis.

Hypertonic solutions   Solutions that draw fluids from cells and tissues across the cell membrane into the bloodstream; an example is 3% normal saline.

Hypotonic solutions   Fluids that move across the cell membrane into surrounding cells and tissues; examples are 0.45% normal saline and 0.3% normal saline.

I

Incompatibility   A chemical, physical, or therapeutic change that occurs when two or more medication or solutions are mixed.

Infectious agent   Pathogen or microorganism that can cause an infection.

Infiltration   The inadvertent administration of a non-vesicant (non-blister-causing) solution or medication into surrounding tissues; occurs when the tip of the IV catheter withdraws from the vein or pokes through the vein.

Infusion pump   Electronically controlled device that provides precise control over the rate of an IV infusion.

Injection cap   A cap placed on the end of a peripheral access device that allows for intermittent IV therapy; also known as a PRN adaptor.

Intake and output (I&O)   A measurement of all the fluids that a patient receives and loses. Examples of intake are oral fluids, fluids from IV infusions, fluids from tube feedings, and any nutrient that is liquid at room temperature. Examples of output are urine, wound suctioning or drainage, and diarrhea.

Intake and output (I&O) record   An area of the medication record that is used to document the patient's intake and output.

Intermittent peripheral infusion device   An IV access site used to administer medications or fluids on a schedule; also known as a saline or heparin lock.

Interstitial fluid (ISF)   Fluid that surrounds the cells

Intracellular fluid (ICF)   Fluid inside the cells.

Intravascular fluid   The fluid in blood; blood plasma

Intravenous (IV)   Within a vein.

Isolation precautions   Steps taken to prevent the spread of infection; some examples are separating the infected patient from others and using personal protective equipment.

Isotonic solutions   Fluids that do not affect the fluid balance of the surrounding cells or tissues; examples are normal saline and lactated ringers.

IV absorbed   Total amount of fluid absorbed by a patient during a shift. This amount is recorded on the intake and output record.

IV flow sheet   An electronic or written record of the amount and type of IV fluid a patient is receiving; also known as an IV administration record, or IV record.

IV to be absorbed (TBA)   Amount of fluid left in the solution container at the time the fluid balance record is totaled.

IVPB   Intravenous piggyback; the administration of IV medications or fluids through a secondary line.

J

Joint Commission on Accreditation of Healthcare Organizations (JCAHO)   A quality oversight body for health care organizations and managed care in the United States.

L

Lumen   The open space in the center of the tube of the catheter.

M

Macrodrip   A type of IV tubing that usually delivers 10 gtt/mL, 15 gtt/mL, or 20 gtt/mL.

Maintenance fluids   IV fluids that are used to maintain the balance of fluids and electrolytes in patients.

MAR   Abbreviation for medication administration record; a written or electronic record of the medications that a patient is receiving.

Mastectomy   Surgical removal of the breast, usually to treat breast cancer.

Microdrip   A type of IV tubing that usually delivers 60 gtt/mL.

Midline catheter   Any catheter placed between the antecubital area and the head of the clavicle.

Milliliter (mL)   A unit of measure in the metric system; used to measure the volume of fluid infused during IV therapy.

mL/h   Milliliters per hour; the flow rate value for most electronically controlled IV infusions.

Mode of transmission   Method by which a pathogen is spread.

N

National Institute of Occupational Safety and Health (NIOSH)   A division of the Centers for Disease Control and Prevention that conducts research and makes recommendations for the prevention of work-related injury and illness.

Needleless systems   IV or phlebotomy systems designed without the need for needles.

Needlestick injuries   Injuries caused by a needle or IV catheter that pierces the skin.

Nosocomial infection   An infection that a patient acquires in a health care facility.

O

Occupation Safety and Health Administration (OSHA)   A division of the U.S. Department of Labor that helps to prevent work-related injuries by coordinating with employers and employees to create a better working environment.

Osmolarity   Concentration of a solution; determines the direction of fluid shift between the extracellular and intracellular compartments.

Osmosis   The transport of fluid across the cell membrane that is dependent on the concentration of solutes in the fluid compartments and stops when the concentrations on both sides of the membrane are equal.

P

Palpate   To examine by touch; to feel.

Parenteral nutrition   The IV infusion of nutrients including amino acids, dextrose, fat, electrolytes, vitamins, and trace elements.

Patient-controlled analgesia (PCA) pump   An electronic device that allows patients to control their own pain medication within limits preset according to the physician's order.

Peripheral IV therapy   The introduction of fluids through a catheter into a vein other than those found in the chest or abdomen; used for short-term therapy.

Peripheral vein   Any vein that is not located on the trunk, head, or neck.

Personal protective equipment   Equipment designed to protect the user, such as masks, gloves, and gowns.

Phlebitis   Irritation and inflammation of the vein caused by mechanical, chemical, or bacterial injury.

Plasma   Fluid portion of the blood.

Plasma expanders   IV fluids that act to expand the intravascular space.

Portal of entry   The method by which a pathogen enters a susceptible host.

Portal of exit   The method by which a pathogen leaves the reservoir.

Precipitate   A solid substance separated from a solution; sediment.

Primary administration set   The main tube for an IV infusion that includes a drip chamber, sterile tube, regulator, and connectors.

PRN adaptor   A cap placed on the end of a peripheral access device that allows for intermittent IV therapy; also known as an injection cap.

R

Rate controller   A type of electronic infusion device that relies on gravity to infuse the solutions, but no clamp is used to adjust the flow rate.

Rehydration   Treatment for fluid loss with IV fluids; also known as fluid replacement.

Replacement fluids   Fluids that replace electrolytes or fluids lost from dehydration, hemorrhage, vomiting, or diarrhea.

Reservoir   The site at which a pathogen grows and multiplies.

Rh system   Blood typing system based on inherited antigens found on the surface of red blood cells; the second most important system for determining blood donor/recipient compatibility.

S

Safe-needle devices   Needles or IV catheters that have safety mechanisms designed to blunt or cover the point.

Saline flush   An injection of saline to flush the intermittent IV line.

Secondary administration set   A small-volume fluid container and administration set used to introduce medication to a patient who has a primary IV in place; also known as a piggyback.

Sepsis   Life-threatening condition as a result of a localized infection; marked by fever, elevated white blood cell count, tachypnea, and tachycardia.

Skin turgor   Elastic properties of the skin, reflecting the body fluid status.

Solutes   Dissolved substances; examples are electrolytes and proteins.

Standard Precautions   Procedures, used with all patients, that are designed to prevent the spread of infection.

Stopcock   A device attached to an IV line that allows for more than one IV fluid to flow into a single IV access device.

Susceptible host   Any person at risk for infection.

Syringe pump   An electronic IV controller used to administer and control smaller amounts of medications.

T

Trocar   The needle inside a cannula used for IV access.

U

Urometer   A specialized urine collection bag with a flow meter.

V

Valves   Structures within the vein that are necessary to keep blood flowing toward the heart and that also allow blood to flow against the force of gravity.

Venipuncture   puncture of a vein with a needle.

Vesicant   A medication or agent that produces blisters.

Virulence   The ability of a pathogen to cause disease.

Volume-control sets   Devices used to improve the accuracy of fluid infusion, especially for small volumes of medication or fluid.

Y

Y set   An IV administration set used for blood transfusions. It is equipped with two short tubes above the drip chamber. One tube is connected to a fluid container of normal saline; the other is connected to the blood. This set typically contains a micron filter.

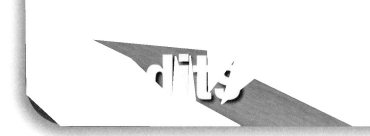

Art Credits

Figures 4.1 a, b, & c: Labels for Lactated Ringer's and 5% Dextrose Injection®; 5% Dextrose Injection®; and 0.9% Sodium Chloride Injection®—Courtesy of Baxter Health Care Corporation. All rights reserved.

Figures 4.4; 8.4a; 8.4b: ©Glaxo Smith Kline. ®FORTAZ is a registered trademark of Glaxo Smith Kline.

Figure 4.5a: Heparin Sodium Injection®—Courtesy of Hospira, Inc., 275 North Field Drive, Lake Forest, IL 60045

Figure 4.5b: ©Copyright Eli Lilly and Company. All rights reserved. Used with permission. ®HUMULIN is a registered trademark of Eli Lilly and Company.

Figure 5.2: Engler—Concepts in Biology, 10/e ©2003, The McGraw-Hill Companies. Reprinted by permission. All right reserved.

Figures 8.3a & 8.3b: Eloxatin®—Courtesy of Sanofi-Aventis.

Photo Credits

Design Elements

(medical icon): © Comstock/Alamy RF; (background image): © Alamy RF; (computer icon): © Corbis RF; (question mark, stethoscope): © PhotoDisc/Getty Images; (caduceus): © Comstock/Alamy RF.

Chapter One

Figure 1.1: © Dynamic Graphics/JupiterImages; **1.3:** © Vol. 72/PhotoDisc/Getty Images; **1.4:** © Vol. 18/PhotoDisc/Getty Images; **1.5:** © Mediscan; **1.6:** © Vol. 106/Corbis; **1.7:** Courtesy of Matt Rhodes.

Chapter Two

Page 25(top to bottom): © Total Care Programming, Inc., Courtesy and © Becton Dickinson, © B. Braun Medical Inc., Courtesy and © Becton Dickinson; **2.2:** Courtesy and © Becton Dickinson; **2.3:** Courtesy and © Becton Dickinson; **2.6:** © The McGraw-Hill Companies, Inc./Jill Braaten, photographer; **2.7:** © The McGraw-Hill Companies, Inc./Jan L. Saeger, photographer; **2.8:** © Total Care Programming, Inc.

Chapter Three

Figure 3.1: © Mediscan; **3.2:** © Getty Royalty Free; **3.4:** Courtesy and © Becton Dickinson; **3.5:** © SGM Photography; **3.6:** Courtesy and © Becton Dickinson; **3.7:** Courtesy of HDC Corporation; **3.8:** © Total Care Programming, Inc.; **3.9:** Courtesy of Kathleen Bell; **3.12a,b:** © Total Care Programming, Inc.; 3.14b: © SGM Photography; 3.16a,b: Courtesy of Estill Medical Technologies; **3.18:** Courtesy of Filtertek, Inc.; **3.19, 3.20:** Courtesy and © Becton Dickinson; **3.21:** © Dynamic Graphics/JupiterImages; **3.22:** © Vol. 18/PhotoDisc/Getty Images; **3.23:** Abbott Labs; **3.25, 3.26, 3.27:** Alaris Medical Systems.

Chapter Four

Figure 4.3: © Antonio Reeve/Photo Researchers.

Chapter Five

Figures 5.1, 5.6: © Total Care Programming, Inc.; **5.8:** Courtesy and © Becton Dickinson.

Chapter Six

Figure 6.2: © Total Care Programming, Inc.; **6.5:** © ER productions/Corbis; **6.6a:** © Mediscan; **6.6b, 6.8a,b:** © Total Care Programming, Inc.; **6.9:** © Mediscan; **6.11:** Courtesy of Venoscope, LLC.

Chapter Seven

Figure 7.1: © Dynamic Graphics/JupiterImages; **7.3, 7.4:** Courtesy of Tycos Health Care; **7.7, 7.8:** © Total Care Programming, Inc.;

Chapter Eight

Figure 8.2: Abbott Labs.

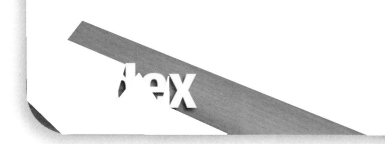

A

Abbreviations
  commonly used for IV solutions, 70
  in documentation, 155–157
  IV fluid abbreviations and concentrations, 201–202
  IV therapy calculations, 206–207
ABO blood groups, 77–78
ABO system, 77
Accessory cephalic vein, 111
Accessory devices of IV administration, 55–57
Active transport, 9
ADD-Vantage system, 191
Administration equipment, 51–52
  accessory devices of IV administration, 55–57
  primary administration sets, 51–54
  secondary administration sets, 52, 54–55
Airborne transmission, infections spread by, 29, 30
Albumin, 76
Alcohol solutions, 77
Aldosterone, 9
Alkylating agents, 91
Allied health personnel, 6
American Association of Medical Assistants (AAMA), 6
Amount to administer (A), 193
Anaphylaxis, 76
Anesthetic cream, 104
Angiocath system, 42
Anions, 8
Answer key, 208–218
Antecubital veins, 41, 109
Antiarrhythmic drugs, 90
Antibiotics, 89
Anticoagulant therapy, 82
Anticoagulants, 90, 166
Anticonvulsants, 91
Antidiuretic hormone (ADH), 9
Antiemetics, 91
Antifungal medications, 89–90
Antihypertensives, 90
Anti-infectives, 88, 89–90
Antimetabolites, 91
Antitumor antibiotics, 91
Antiulcer medications, 91
Antiviral medications, 90
Anxiolytic agents, 91
Aseptic technique, 109

B

Bags, IV fluid, 57–58
Basilic vein, 111
Bicarbonate infusions, 76
Blanching, 139
Bleeding prevention, after discontinuation of an IV, 167
Blood and blood products, 77, 78
  ABO blood groups, 77–78
  administering, 10–12
  blood transfusions, 80
  compatible blood groups, 77, 79
  labeled, 135
  Rh factor, 79–80
Blood-borne pathogens, 22
Blood components, 77, 79
Blood plasma, 8
Blood transfusions, 11–12, 80
Blunt cannula and resealable ports, 26
Body fluids, 7–8
Bronchospasm, 143
Broviac catheter, 16, 47, 48
Butterfly (catheter/needle), 43

C

Calcium, 8
Calculations, IV therapy, 173
  conversions, abbreviations, and formulas for, 206–207
  flow rates, 173–183
  infusion time and volume, 184–190
  intermittent infusions, 191–196
  preventing malpractice, 173
Calibration factor, 177
Cannula systems, 43
Cannulation, 107, 114
Capillary filtration, 9
Capillary reabsorption, 9
Cardiovascular medications, 88, 90
Caring for IV patients, 130–131
  common problems and solutions, 145–148
  complications and risks, 138–144
  labeling, 131–135
  monitoring the IV site, 141, 158–160
  review, 149–151
  site dressings and changes, 136–138
Catheters and access devices, 40
  catheter sizes, 50–51
  central IV therapy catheters, 15–16
  needleless systems, 44–49
  peripheral access devices, 41–43

Cations, 8
Centers for Disease Control and Prevention (CDC), 3
  hand hygiene, 32
  isolation precautions, 31
  Standard Precautions, 31
  use of gloves, 33
Central IV therapy, 14–16
Central nervous system medications, 88, 90–91
Central venous catheters, 46
Central venous lines, 16
Centrally placed external catheters, 46–48
Centrally placed internal ports, 48–49
Cephalic vein, 111
Certified medical assistant (CMA), 6
Chain of infection, 29–30
Chemical incompatibility, 85
Chemotherapeutic agents, 88, 91–92
Children. See Pediatric patients
Chloride, 8
Closed IV system, maintaining a, 57
Commission on Accreditation of Allied Health Education Programs (CAAHEP), Standards and Guidelines for Medical Assisting Educational Programs, 6
Compatibility, IV solution, 85–86
Competency checklists, 219–227
Complications and risks from IV therapy, 138
  extravasation, 140–141
  infiltration, 138–140
  other complications, 143–144
  phlebitis, 141–143
Congestive heart failure, 90
Congestive heart failure agents, 90
Consent for IV therapy, 12
Contact transmission, infections spread by, 30
Conversions for IV calculations, 206
Cycle-nonspecific agents, 91
Cycle-specific agents, 91

D

Department of Labor, U.S., 3
Desired dose (D), 192
Dextran, 76
Dextrose solutions, 75
  sodium chloride and, 71, 74, 75
Diffusion, 9
Digital dorsal veins, 110

Discontinuing an IV, 165–167
Diuretics, 90
Documenting and discontinuation, 152–153
  abbreviations in documentation, 155–157
  discontinuing an IV, 165–167
  documentation after IV discontinuation, 154–155
  documentation after IV initiation, 153
  documentation during IV therapy, 154, 155
  documentation recommendations, 155
  documenting fluid balance, 161–165
  documenting IV problems, 158–160
  documenting IV therapy, 153–158
  monitoring IV therapy, 158–160
  review, 169–171
Dorsal metacarpal veins, 111
Dosage unit (Q), 192
Dose on hand (H), 192
Double lumen PICC, 15, 45
Dressings. See Site dressings and changes
Drop factor, 176
Droplet transmission, infections spread by, 29, 30
Drops per minute (gtt/min), 173, 174, 176–180

E

Ecchymosis, 147
Elderly patients. See Geriatric patients
Electrolytes, 8–9
  electrolyte solutions, 73, 74, 76
  and vitamins, 83–84
Electronic flow control devices, 59
EMLA, 104
Erythema, 141
Extension tubing, 54
Extracellular fluid (ECF), 8, 70, 73
Extravasation, 87, 140–141
Eye protection, 33, 34

F

Face shields, 34
Fear of needles, patient, 103
Filters, 55–56
Flash, 119
Flow rates, 52–53, 145–147
Flow rates, calculating, 173–174
  adjusting flow rates, 181–183
  in drops per minute (gtt/min), 176–180
  in milliliters per hour (mL/h), 174–176
  recalculating flow rates, 183
Flow sheet, 105, 113, 164
Fluid and electrolyte balance
  electrolytes, 8–9
  fluid movement, 9
  maintaining, 7–9
  other fluid regulation processes, 9
  fluid bags, 57–59

Fluid balance, documenting, 161
  documenting fluids, 162–165
  intake and output, 161
Fluid replacement, 101
Food and Drug Administration (FDA), U.S., 22

G

Gastrointestinal medications, 88, 91
Gauges, catheter, 50–51
Generic drugs, 87–88
Geriatric patients
  fluid and electrolyte balance in, 10
  fluid and electrolyte disorders in, 84
  IV insertions in, 122–123
Glossary, 228–231
Gloves, 33–34
Goggles, 34
Gowns, 34, 103–104
Gravity drip, 59
Gravity infusion, 59
Groshong catheters, 46–47

H

Hand hygiene, 32–33
Health Insurance Portability and Accountability Act (HIPAA), 3, 6, 162
Heart failure, 90
Hematomas, 147
Hemolytic reaction, 77
Heparin, 82
Heparin flush, 42–43, 48
Heparin lock, 192
Hepatitis B virus (HBV), 22
Hepatitis C virus (HCV), 22
Hetastarch, 76
Hickman catheter, 15, 47, 48
High-alert medication, 93
Hinged-recap, needle, 25
Hormones, fluid regulation and, 8, 9
Human immunodeficiency virus (HIV), 22
Hypersensitivity reaction, 143
Hypertonic solutions, 72, 73
Hypotonic solutions, 72, 73

I

Immobilization, 123–124
Implantable ports, 16
Incidence report, 143
Incompatibility, IV solution, 85
Infection control, 21, 22, 28
  chain of infection, 29–30
  hand hygiene, 32–33
  modes of transmission, 30
  personal protective equipment, 33–35
  preventing infections, 30–35
Infectious agents, 29
Infiltration, 60, 76–77, 139–140
Infusion Nurses Society, 117
Infusion pumps, 60–61, 63, 114, 146
Infusion time, calculating, 184–188
Infusion volume, calculating, 184, 188–190

Injection cap, 42, 56
INS Infiltration Scale, 139, 140
INS Phlebitis Scale, 142
Insulin, 83
Intake and output (I&O), 161
Intake and output (I&O) record, 162–163
Intermittent infusions, calculating, 191, 196
  intermittent peripheral infusion devices, 191–192
  preparing and calculating intermittent infusions, 192–195
  preventing errors, 195
  secondary lines (piggyback), 191
Intermittent peripheral infusion devices, 191–192
Interstitial fluid (ISF), 8
Intracellular fluid (ICF), 8, 70
Intramuscular (IM) administration, 10, 87
Intravascular fluid (IVF), 8
Intravenous (IV) fluids, 57–59, 69–72
  abbreviations for, 70, 155–157, 201–202, 206–207
  additives, 80–84
  common IV medications, 74, 86–94, 204–205
  compatibility, 85–86
  incompatible IV solutions, 203
  IV fluid bags, 57–59
  labels, 71
  review, 96–98
  types and uses of, 72–80
Intravenous (IV) therapy calculations, 172–173
  adjusting flow rates, 181–183
  calculating flow rates, 173–180
  calculating infusion time and volume, 184–190
  calculating intermittent infusions, 191–196
  conversions, abbreviations, and formulas for, 206–207
  preventing malpractice, 173
  review, 198–200
Intravenous (IV) therapy practices, 1–2
  allied health personnel, 6
  intravenous defined, 2
  medical assistants, 6
  reasons for IV therapy, 7–13
  and regulation, 3–5
  review, 18–20
  roles and responsibilities, 5–7
  types of IV therapy, 13–16
Intravenous (IV) therapy supplies and equipment, 39–40
  administration equipment, 51–57
  catheters and access devices, 40–49
  fluids, 57–59
  IV regulators, 59–64
  review, 65–68
  venous access device selection, 49–51
Isolation precautions, 31
Isotonic solutions, 72–73
IV absorbed, 164

IV access, 145
IV flow sheet, 105, 113, 164
IV fluid bags, 57–59
IV medications, common, 86–87,
   204–205
   administration of IV medications,
      10, 87, 92–93
   anti-infectives, 89–90
   cardiovascular medications, 90
   central nervous system medications,
      90–91
   chemotherapeutic agents, 91–92
   classification of medications, 87–92
   gastrointestinal medications, 91
   incompatible medications and
      solutions, 203
   medication errors, 94
   preparing IV medication, 106
IV piggyback (IVPB), 84, 191
IV poles, 57
IV regulators, 59
   infusion pumps, 60–61
   manual monitoring, 59–60
   patient-controlled analgesia pumps,
      61–62
   rate controllers, 61
   syringe pumps, 61
   volume-control sets, 62–63
IV removal problems, 147
IV to be absorbed (TBA), 164

J

Joint Commission on Accreditation
   of Healthcare Organizations
   (JCAHO), 3, 153, 156

K

Ketoacidosis, 76, 83
KVO infusions, 52

L

Labeling, 131–132
   IV fluid bag labels, 58, 133, 134
   pharmacy label, 134
   rate label, 133–134
   site label, 131, 133
Licensed practical nurses (LPNs), 6
Licensed vocational nurses (LVNs), 6
Long-term IV therapy, 49
Luer-activated devices (LADs), 26–27
Lumen, 15, 43, 45

M

Macrodrip tubing, 52, 53, 176–177
Magnesium, 8, 84
Maintenance fluids, 76
Mannitol, 76
MAR (medication administration
   record), 105
Masks, 33, 34
Mastectomy, 106
Measures for IV calculations, 206
Median antebrachial vein, 111

Median cephalic and median basilic
   veins, 111
Medical assistants (MAs), 6
Medication errors, 94
Medications. See IV medications,
   common
MediPort, 48
Metabolic acidosis, 76
Microdrip tubing, 52, 53, 177
Midline catheters, 44–45
Milliliter (mL), 52
Milliliters per hour (mL/h), 173, 174–176
Mode of transmission (chain of
   infection), 29–30
Monitoring and maintaining IV
   therapy. See Caring for IV patients
Multiple electrolyte solutions, 76

N

Narcotic analgesics, 91
National Healthcare Quality Report,
   2003, 22
National Institute of Occupational
   Safety and Health (NIOSH), 3, 22
National Patient Safety Standards
   (JCAHO), 3, 4
Needleless syringes, 44
Needleless systems, 22, 24, 26–28, 44
   central venous catheters, 46
   centrally placed external catheters,
      46–48
   midline peripheral catheters and
      peripherally inserted central
      catheters, 15–16, 44–45
Needles
   recapping, 124
   and syringes, 41–42
Needlestick injuries, 22, 23
Needlestick Safety and Prevention
   Act, 3, 5, 22
Nitrosoureas, 91
Noninvasive procedures, IV therapy, 6
Nosocomial infections, 30–31
Nurse Practice Act, 6
Nutrients and nutritional
   supplements, delivering, 12

O

Obese patients, IV insertions in, 123
Occupational Safety and Health
   Administration (OSHA), 3, 5
   safety standards for needle
      devices, 43
   sharps injury protection rules, 44
Osmolarity, 70–71, 73
Osmosis, 9
Over-the-needle catheter, 42–43

P

Palpate, 109
Parenteral nutrition, 12, 80–82
Patient-care technicians (PCTs), 6
Patient-controlled analgesia (PCA)
   pumps, 61–62

Patient identification and screening,
   105
   screening and monitoring during IV
      administration, 106
   screening before an IV infusion,
      105–106
Patient preparation for IV infusion,
   102
   changing a gown, 104
   establishing patient contact, 102
   physical preparation, 103–104
   psychological preparation, 103
Patient privacy, 16, 102
Pediatric patients
   fluid and electrolyte balance in, 10
   IV insertions in, 123–124
Peripheral access devices
   needle and syringe, 41–42
   over-the-needle catheter, 42–43
   steel needle, 43
Peripheral IV therapy, 13–14
   initiation of, 116–122
   peripheral veins, 108–110
   site selection, 107–112
Peripheral parenteral nutrition (PPN), 81
Peripheral veins, 41, 108–112
Peripherally inserted central catheter
   (PICC), 15–16, 44–45
Personal protective equipment (PPE),
   33–35
Pharmacy label, 134
Phenytoin, 91
Phlebitis, 87, 141–143
Phosphate, 8
Phosphorus, 84
Physical incompatibility, 85
Physical preparation, for IV infusion,
   103–104
Physician's orders, for IV therapy
   initiation, 101–102
Piggyback (IVPB), 191
Piggyback set, 54
Plasma, 77
Plasma expanders, 76–77
Plastic IV fluid bags, 57–58
Port-a-Cath, 48
Portal of entry (chain of infection), 30
Portal of exit (chain of infection), 29
Potassium, 8, 84
Precipitate, 84
Preparation for the IV infusion, 99–104
   changing a gown, 104
   establishing patient contact, 102
   initiation of peripheral IV therapy,
      116–122
   patient identification and screening,
      105–107
   patient preparation, 102
   physical preparation, 103–104
   physician's orders, 101–102
   preparation of supplies and
      equipment, 112–116
   psychological preparation, 103
   review, 126–129
   site selection for peripheral IVs,
      107–112
   special populations, 122–125

Pressure-activated safety valve devices, 27–28
Primary administration sets, 51–54
Privacy, patient, 16, 102
PRN adaptors, 42, 56
Problems with IV therapy
  flow rates, 145–147
  IV access, 145
  IV removal problems, 147
Protective sheath/cap, needle, 25, 121
Psychological preparation, for IV infusion, 103

R

Rate controllers, 61
Rate label, 133–134
Recapping needles, 124
Registered medical assistant (RMA), 6
Registered nurses (RNs), 6
Regulators. *See* IV regulators
Rehydration, 101
Replacement fluids, 76
Reservoir (chain of infection), 29
Retractable needle, 25
Rh factor, 79–80
Rh system, 79
Roller clamps, 53

S

Safe-needle and needleless devices, 22–23
  needleless systems, 24, 26–28
  safe-needle devices, 22, 23–24, 25
Safety and infection control, 21–22
  infection control, 28–35
  review, 36–38
  standards for safe-needle and needleless devices, 22–28
Safety clip, needle, 25
Saline flush, 42, 48
Saline lock, 192
Screening procedure
  before an IV infusion, 105–106
  screening and monitoring during IV administration, 106

Screw clamps, 53
Secondary administration sets, 52, 54–55, 191
Secondary lines (piggyback), 191
Sedatives, 91
Self-blunting needle, 25
Sepsis, 143
Short-term IV therapy, 13
Single lumen PICC, 15, 45
Site dressings and changes, 136, 138
  caring for the IV site, 136–137
  changing the dressing, 137
Site label, 131, 133
Skin turgor, 122
Slide clamps, 53
Sodium, 8
Sodium bicarbonate solution, 76
Sodium chloride solutions, 71, 74, 75
  dextrose and, 71, 74, 75
Solutes, 7–8
Special populations, 122–125
Standard Precautions, 31, 34, 144
Standards and Guidelines for Medical Assisting Educational Programs (CAAHEP), 6
Steel needle, 43
Stopcock, 56
Subcutaneous (sub-Q) administration, 10, 87
Supplies and equipment, for IV infusion, 112–116
Susceptible host (chain of infection), 30
Syringe and needle device, 41
Syringe pumps, 61
Syringes, needleless, 44

T

Therapeutic incompatibility, 85
Thirst, 9
Total parenteral nutrition (TPN), 81–82
Trade names, medication, 87, 88
Transfusion reaction, 78
Trocar, 43
Tunneled catheters, 47–48

U

Universal donor, 77
Universal Precautions, 31
Universal recipient, 77
Urometer, 161

V

Valves, 109
Vasodilators, 90
Vector-borne (chain of infection), 30
Vehicle-borne transmission, infections spread by, 29, 30
Venipuncture sites, 109, 124
Venous access device selection, 49–51, 122
Vesicant drugs, 140–141
Vinca alkaloids, 91
Virulence (chain of infection), 29
Vitamins, and electrolytes, 83–84
Volume-control sets, 62–63

W

Washing, hand, 32–33
Water, 9
White blood cell transfusions, 11
Wing-tipped (butterfly) catheter, 43
Wrapping technique (immobilization), 123–124

Y

Y set, 54, 55